Dysautonomia, POTS Syndrome

Diagnosis, symptoms, treatment, causes, doctors, nervous disorders, prognosis, research, history, diet, physical therapy, medication, environment, and more all covered!

By Frederick Earlstein

Foreword

Let me get one thing off the table immediately. I am not a doctor. My experience with POTS began when my only niece started to have unexplained fainting spells just after she turned 14.

I watched with growing frustration while my sister and her family went through doctor after doctor after doctor. It seemed as if every day a new email appeared in my InBox describing the latest test the doctors forced Sylvie to endure.

There were frightening "diagnoses" that turned out to be wrong within days, never mind the agony the family suffered in those long hours before some doctor basically said, "Oh. Sorry. Wrong!"

It was scary, maddening, and needless to say made us all less than respectful in our attitude toward the medical community. Over a period of months, everyone in the extended family started searching the net for Sylvie's strange symptoms as the poor child got sicker and sicker.

In truth she was getting more and more terrified of what would happen if she stood up, and in no time was being home schooled and had no social life beyond the contacts she maintained online. The once sunny, happy young woman was clearly depressed and miserable.

Finally the acronym "POTS" came into the discussion. Research links started flying and my sister put the question to Sylvie's pediatrician. Thankfully, he was open to reading the information and then acted on what he learned. That got the ball rolling, and we learned — to our immense relief — that she would likely grow out of her symptoms in time.

I found myself envious of some of the recommendations she received to improve her condition. I struggle with maintaining a normal blood pressure level and Sylvie was being told to eat more salt! One dietary guide recommendation suggested she have a "shot" of pickle juice each morning. (That I could do without.)

After changing her diet and beginning a program of exercise to overcome the "deconditioning" that resulted from her time at home, which was largely spent reclining, Sylvie is doing very well. There were also some necessary accommodations at school, but I'm happy to say that once the administrators understood the nature of her illness, they were very helpful.

Sylvie must stay well hydrated and have salty snacks throughout the day, and in the beginning only attended afternoon classes since mornings were tough on her — but now she is back on campus and thrilled to be with her friends again.

The information that I've compiled in this book is based on my own notes and reading over the several months it took for Sylvie to be accurately diagnosed. Certainly it's all out there on the Internet, but piecing it together is time consuming and frustrating. I hope this text will offer you a shortcut that will lead to better questions and a faster diagnosis for your own loved one. Waiting out long months of trial and error is demoralizing, and the patient can lose a lot of ground in that time.

POTS research is ongoing, so there will be changes — hopefully positive ones — in the near future. Already researchers are exploring the potential for an autoimmune basis for POTS and more attention is being paid to its genetic links.

I've chosen to include a chapter on medical terms — you'll be slammed with a lot of them — and the text is littered with links to useful sites online and even blogs that contain first-person accounts of life with POTS.

(Just so those links don't get lost in the shuffle, I've rounded them up and included them in a "Relevant Websites" section at the back of the book along with other useful online resources I've located.)

I've tried to help you understand that in Sylvie's case we were dealing with developmental POTS, but the condition can be linked to many different diseases. POTS itself isn't an illness, but rather a symptom of a larger problem.

Hopefully I've simplified, but not committed the crime of dumbing down. Frankly, the doctors rather expect us to be dumb. That's the weakest position you can adopt in dealing with the medical community. Get educated, get informed, and never stop asking questions! You are your own best health advocate, and certainly the best advocate for your child!

I'd like to say this is a definitive look at POTS, but that would be pretty arrogant. Instead, I'll say I've tried to give you as complete a picture as I can based on my own research. I promise you'll be better off than I was starting with zero comprehension and motivated by concern for my kid sister and my niece.

I sincerely wish you all good luck on your own personal path with POTS. The condition isn't fatal, but it is life-changing, and, like many "invisible" illnesses POTS is greatly misunderstood. But one thing is certainly clear to the POTS patient — something is very wrong!

Acknowledgments

I would like to express my gratitude towards my family, friends, and colleagues for their kind co-operation and encouragement which helped me in completion of this book.

My thanks and appreciations go to my colleagues and people who have willingly helped me out with their abilities.

In addition, I would like to make a very special dedication of this book to my niece, Sylvie, who inspired this project and is a remarkable young lady. Love Always!

Acknowledgments

Table of Contents

Table of Contents

Table of Contents

Table of Contents

Part 1 - POTS and Associated Disorders

A person first coming to grips with a diagnosis of POTS (Postural Orthostatic Tachycardia Syndrome) enters a world of confusing and overlapping symptoms, conditions, terminology and acronyms.

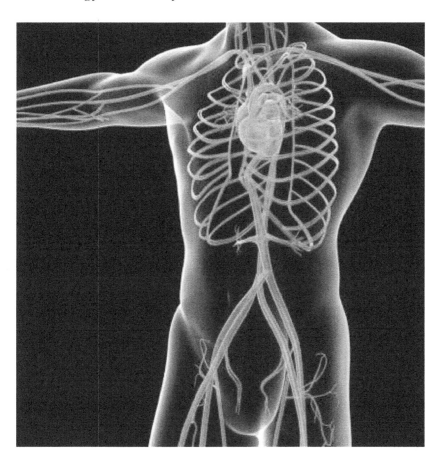

It's common to hear the words "POTS" and "dysautonomia" used interchangeably. Technically, dysautonomia is an umbrella term for several malfunctions of the autonomic nervous system including POTS.

As we will explore in greater detail in Part 3, the autonomic nervous systems controls those bodily functions that do not require conscious thought. Things like heart rate, blood pressure, and digestion stay on "auto pilot" as we go about our day-to-day lives.

People who live with some form of dysautonomia become unusually aware of these systems when they experience the negative effects of poor circulation, abnormal blood pressure, or a high heart rate.

In the case of POTS, this awareness becomes triggered by the simple act of standing up. The autonomic nervous system improperly controls the reaction of the body to the gravitational pull of standing and adverse symptoms result, including, but not limited to, fainting.

Estimates suggest that more than 25 million people around the world deal with some kind of dysautonomia. None are "curable" per se, but all can be managed or improved once a correct diagnosis is made, often through dietary changes or environmental modifications.

In isolation, POTS is most often a condition seen in young people, usually after an intense growth spurt. To distinguish this variant from other types, it is generally referred to as "Developmental POTS." Many such cases resolve over time with the help of correct supportive strategies.

However, POTS can also manifest due to other causes and in connection with other conditions, greatly complicating both treatment and management.

Unfortunately, there is not only a lack of public awareness about the various forms of dysautonomia, but also a shocking level of misunderstanding among doctors themselves. Many POTS patients, especially young people, experience years of endless rounds of tests only to be told they have a psychological problem.

Developmental POTS is one of the most prevalent forms of dysautonomia. It is believed to affect 1 out of 100 teenagers. This means in America alone, there could be 500,000 to 3,000,000 people at any one time dealing with a host of symptoms that include, but are not limited to:

- lightheadedness
- fainting
- tachycardia (racing heart rate)
- chest pains
- shortness of breath
- gastrointestinal upset
- shaking
- exercise intolerance
- temperature sensitivity

Young women are most likely to suffer from Developmental POTS and to grapple with a level of disability comparable to that seen in COPD and congestive heart failure. The severity of their symptoms increases markedly during menstruation when their overall blood volume drops.

Thankfully most cases of Developmental POTS resolve over a period of time. Supportive measures involving diet and lifestyle are typically effective and fairly simple to put into place.

The condition can exist in concert with many other illnesses, however, including diabetes, multiple sclerosis, rheumatoid arthritis, celiac, Sjogren's syndrome, lupus, and Parkinson's, and thus may affect almost anyone at any time in their lives.

Along with POTS, the two other most common forms of dysautonomia are Neurocardiogenic Syncope (NCS) and Multiple System Atrophy (MSA). NCS causes one or two fainting spells over the course of a person's life. In severe cases however, the patient faints several times per day. This increases their risk for broken bones and even traumatic brain injury. The patient's ability to work, attend school, or engage in social activities is severely compromised.

MSA is a fatal neurodegenertive disorder similar to Parkinson's disease that occurs in adults age 40 and up. Within 2 years of diagnosis, a patient with MSA is typically bedridden. Most die within 5-10 years. MSA is rare, currently affecting approximately 350,000 patients worldwide.

POTS Overview

POTS or Postural Orthostatic Tachycardia Syndrome refers

to an abnormal increase in heart rate relative to posture.

People with POTS experience "orthostatic intolerance," or adverse reactions when standing upright from a sitting or horizontal position. Severity varies from feeling weak or lightheaded, to actual dizziness and fainting within 10 minutes, a symptom called "syncope."

In chronic cases, a POTS patient may not be able to stand or walk for even brief periods, a disability potentially complicated by the concurrent presence of low blood pressure (hypotension.)

Although the medical definition of POTS is straightforward, the syndrome is not as simplistic as it might appear on first blush, which we will explore throughout this text.

The specific criteria for a diagnosis of POTS is the experience of a heart rate increase of 30-40 beats per minute (bpm) upon standing, or having a standing heart rate of more than 120 bpm. These symptoms must continue for more than six months.

Diagnosis may be difficult, however, since POTS is rarely the first condition considered. Patients go through rounds of testing looking for other causes due in large part to the widespread unawareness of POTS in the broader medical community.

Once POTS is correctly identified, however, it can be treated or managed. If the cause is developmental in nature, the symptoms often disappear over time. POTS is not a deadly condition, but it can be a life-altering one even in the short term.

Brief History

The acronym POTS was coined in 1993 by a team of researchers at the Mayo Clinic led by Dr. Phillip A. Low, Professor of Neurology.* Over the past 150 years, multiple labels have been used for the disorder to which this shorthand refers, including, but not limited to:

- **DaCosta's Syndrome** – This name is in tribute to Jacob Mendes Da Costa who described and studied the disorder during the American Civil War.

- **Soldier's Heart** – The name "Soldier's Heart" was the colloquial name for Da Costa's Syndrome, also dating to the United States in the 1860s.

- **Mitral Valve Prolapse Syndrome** – This is an extant syndrome in which the valve separating the upper and lower chambers on the left side of the heart does not function appropriately. It may cause POTS-like symptoms, but it is not the cause of POTS as it is understood in modern terms.

- **Neurocirculatory Asthenia** – The term "neurocirculatory asthenia" replaced "DeCostas's Syndrome" in popular usage during the First World War. During the same time period, the British referred to the condition as "Effort Syndrome."

- **Chronic Orthostatic Intolerance** – Chronic orthostatic intolerance is a phrase you will still see used today, especially in relation to chronic fatigue syndrome. It is descriptively accurate in that it means a person has an ongoing intolerance to standing or being upright without experiencing negative symptoms.

- **Orthostatic Tachycardia** – Orthostatic tachycardia is also used to describe instances of rapid heartbeat when a person moves from a reclining or sitting position to an upright one.

- **Postural Tachycardia Syndrome** – Postural Tachycardia Syndrome is the phrase from which the acronym POTS is derived. It has been in popular use since 1993.

* Dr. Low remains a leading researcher in the field of human autonomic dysfunction, orthostatic intolerance, and postural tachycardia syndrome. Please see Part 5 for a partial listing of his more recent academic publications on the subject.

Once regarded as a psychological condition, POTS is now understood to be a malfunction of the autonomic nervous system with multiple potential causes. Technically it is a "nervous condition," but not in a psychological sense.

In the most abbreviated terms, a person with POTS experiences an abnormal increase in heart rate on standing from a seated position or from lying down.

The resulting effects are similar to instances of low blood pressure, however, the patient's BP may remain stable. Some of the likely symptoms include:

- dizziness
- fainting, often within 10 minutes of standing
- headache
- sweating
- tremors or "shakiness"
- nausea
- brain "fog" / poor concentration
- discoloration in the hands and feet
- chest pains

Anxiety is not the direct cause of POTS, but the patient may develop anxiety out of fear over what might happen when they stand. This nervousness often must be addressed as part of the treatment because it makes patients reluctant to continue to engage in daily activities, leading many to become sedentary or even bedridden.

Depression often results from this dramatic change in quality of life, creating a vicious psychological cycle that is often mistaken for the primary illness rather than being recognized as a psychological complication of the underlying disorder.

Researchers now understand POTS can take multiple forms, leading to increased sophistication in both diagnostic and treatment protocols in just the last 20 years.

Classifications of POTS

The following classifications are applied to POTS. The designations may refer to identified causes of the syndrome, or to the manner in which the symptoms present.

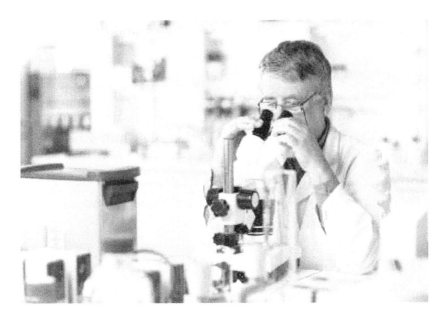

High / Low Flow

This system focuses on irregularities in peripheral blood blow and peripheral arterial resistance. The three designated groups are:

(Please note the abbreviation Pv stands for pulmonary venous pressure. Pulmonary circulation carries deoxygenated blood away from the heart and to the lungs for oxygenation before returning the blood to the heart.)

Low Blood Flow, High Arterial Resistance, High-Pv

Defects in local blood flow regulation and mild absolute hypovolemia (decreased volume of circulating blood) cause "Low Flow POTS." Recent research ties this condition to reduced levels of neuronal nitric oxide (nNOS).

Normal Blood Flow, Arterial Resistance, and Pv

In this group, patients have normal peripheral resistance when reclining that becomes "enhanced" upon standing. Venous pooling, the accumulation of blood due to gravitational pool, is observed in the splanchnic vascular bed.
(Splanchnic circulation consists of three vascular beds. Together they are comprised of the stomach, pancreas, small intestine, and colon.)

High Blood Flow, Low Arterial Resistance, Normal-to-Decreased Pv

In "High Flow POTS," inadequate peripheral vasoconstriction (contraction or narrowing of the blood vessels) when lying down or standing leads to high cardiac output, the amount of blood pumping through the circulatory system per minute.

Developmental POTS

Developmental POTS most often affects teenagers age 12-14 after a rapid growth surge. Symptoms worsen until age 16, and in 80% of cases disappear by age 19-24. Researchers have not identified a definitive cause for this developmental variant.

Deconditioning

"Deconditioning" refers to being out of shape after an injury or illness necessitating prolonged bed rest. Inefficient heart function triggers the symptoms when the person stands up. In turn, patients don't attempt exercise to avoid the negative reaction, worsening both their level of deconditioning and their orthostatic symptoms.

Classification by Primary Symptoms

Other classifying terminology used with POTS include:

- hypovolemic, associated with low blood volume

- partial dysautonomic or neuropathic, associated with a partial autonomic neuropathy (damage to the autonomic nerves)

  This form of POTS begins suddenly following a viral illness, pregnancy, surgery, trauma, or a course of immunizations.

- hyperadrenergic, associated with elevated levels of norepinephrine and a rise in systolic blood pressure when standing

  This form is much less common and can be mistaken for an adrenaline-producing tumor, which should be diagnostically ruled out.

Who Develops POTS?

Although anyone can develop POTS, the syndrome is most often seen in healthy women (75-80% of cases) between the ages of 14 and 50. Research has identified a genetic component within some families.

Even given this profile, however, POTS can present as a sudden onset syndrome in the aftermath of an acute illness, an experience of trauma, exposure to toxins.
POTS can overlap other diseases and syndromes. In these cases, resolving the underlying condition does not always eradicate the POTS symptoms.

Some initial causes or complications to be ruled out include prolonged deconditioning from illness, chronic dehydration, diabetic neuropathy, and negative drug reactions. Particular care should be taken with diuretics and blood pressure medications.

What Causes POTS?

The question, "What causes POTS?" is the most difficult to answer, and is a topic that will be taken up in greater detail in Part 3. This "heterogeneous" syndrome (one with many causes) can be seen as part of a group of disorders with similar clinical manifestations.

For this reason, patients must understand that POTS is not a disease, but rather a cluster of symptoms pointing to different causal agents. Identifying those causes in each patient is the greatest challenge of dealing with a diagnosis of POTS. In some cases, doctors are forced to declare the case idiopathic, meaning "of unknown origin."

The conditions listed in the next section are some of the illnesses doctors may seek to rule out in arriving at a clinical explanation for POTS-like symptoms. I am not attempting an encyclopedic explanation of these illnesses.

The following material is only a brief overview of each since they may come up in consultations with doctors and can be the explanation for the symptoms a patient is experiencing.

Clearly if any of these illnesses is diagnosed, patients and their families should immediately learn as much as possible about the illness, its effects, complications, and treatment.

Statistical Overview of POTS

According to the Mayo Clinic, the following statistics are true of POTS and POTS patients:

- Approximately 75% of those affected are women. Of those 75-80% are of menstruating age.

- Women are 5 times more likely than men to develop POTS.

- POTS affects approximately 1 out of every 100 teenagers.

- At least 50% of cases involve some abnormal and often degenerative state of the nervous system (neuropathy/neuropathic.)

- Approximately 1 out of 7 cases shows evidence of an autoimmune component.

- One study determined that of 152 POTS patients, 12.5% had a family member with a similar history of orthostatic intolerance.

- Approximately one-third of POTS patients also present with digestive problems.

- In 1999, an estimated 500,000 people in the United States were dealing with POTS.*

It is extremely difficult to arrive at a workable estimate of how many people suffer from POTS. The upsurge in research in the past 20 years has led to more accurate diagnoses, but total population numbers are still very sketchy and vary widely.

Associated / Related Nervous Disorders

Cultivating a broader understanding of POTS means understanding, at least in a peripheral way, the disorders and conditions that are often concurrent with the syndrome and its symptoms. These include, but are not limited to the following:

Amyloidosis

"Amyloidosis" does not refer to a single disease, but rather to a group of disorders. All involve abnormal groupings of proteins fibers in tissues called amyloid deposits, which break down at a very slow rate. The deposits can occur anywhere in the body or may be localized to one organ or tissue type where they alter structural components and interfere with function.

Thirty different proteins can accumulate in this fashion, but not all are linked to significant disease. Each protein type presents with a different clinical picture and set of symptoms specific to the affected region. Variation among patients can be considerable.

Two of the most common are associated with underlying conditions and are systemic (affecting the whole body). The first of these, AL amyloidosis, is seen most often with non-malignant bone marrow disorders.

AL can, however, also be present in multiple myeloma (bone cancer) cases. The second, AA amyloidosis is present with some type of chronic inflammation like rheumatoid arthritis.

No specific anti-amyloid drugs are available outside the laboratory setting. Treatment focuses on stabilizing organ function. Often the deposits do diminish over time when the underlying condition responds to treatment.

Autoimmune Autonomic Ganglionopathy

The rare condition Autoimmune Autonomic Ganglionopathy (AAG) causes the body to damage receptors in the autonomic ganglia of peripheral nerve fibers. AAG is a treatable disorder than can affect males and females regardless of age. About one-third of patients experience spontaneous improvement, but with incomplete recovery. Onset may be acute, subacute, or gradual and the course of the disease is variable.

Symptoms may include:

- severe low blood pressure upon standing
- fainting
- constipation and associated gastrointestinal issues
- urinary retention
- fixed and dilated pupils
- dry mouth and eyes

Many of these symptoms are POTS like, but no clear link exists between the two conditions. The rarity of AAG has not led to any extensive clinical trials to determine optimal treatment protocols.

Diabetes

Although most people are aware of diabetes in a peripheral sense, few understand the mechanism underlying this common disease. The food that we eat is broken down into blood glucose, a form of sugar, which is the body's primary source of fuel.

After food is digested, the glucose produced passes into the blood stream and is distributed among the body's cells where it is used as energy and for growth. For glucose to enter the cells, however, insulin, a hormone produced by the pancreas, must also be present.

When diabetes develops, the pancreas make too little or too much insulin, or the cells are unable to respond to the insulin that is produced. Glucose builds up in the blood and is then lost in large doses via the urine. The body derives no energy benefit under these circumstances.

The three types of diabetes are Type 1, Type 2, and gestational. Type 1 is an autoimmune disease. The body's immune system destroys the beta cells in the pancreas that produce insulin. Patients with this form of the disease must take insulin daily.

Type 1 develops most often in children, but can appear at any age. Symptoms include excessive thirst, frequent urination, constant hunger, blurred vision, extreme fatigue, and weight loss. If left untreated, the patient may lapse into a fatal diabetic coma.

Type 2 is the most common, affecting 90-95% of diagnosed diabetic cases. It is associated with aging, obesity, and physical inactivity. This form of the disease has both genetic and ethnic links (African American, Mexican American, and Pacific Islander.)

Although insulin is being produced, the body is insulin resistant and does not effectively use the hormone. Symptoms, if present, include fatigue, thirst, hunger, frequent urination, slow healing of wounds, blurred vision, and weight loss.

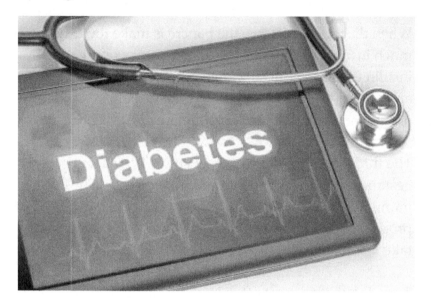

Gestational diabetes develops late in pregnancy and disappears after the child is born. A reasonable body weight and being physically active are good preventive measures. The condition surfaces in 3-8% of pregnancies in the United States. Like Type 2, gestational diabetes has genetic and ethnic links.

Sjogren's Syndrome

The autoimmune disorder Sjogren's often appears alongside other autoimmune conditions including rheumatoid arthritis and lupus. It affects the mucous membranes and moisture-secreting glands of the eyes and mouth causing chronic dryness.

In most cases, patients are 40 years or older at the time of diagnosis. The condition is more common in women, with treatment focusing on symptom relief. The eyes burn and itch, with a sandy, gritty sensation, while the mouth feels stuffed with cotton, to the point that swallowing and speaking become difficult.

Additional symptoms may include:

- painful, swollen and/or stiff joints
- swollen salivary glands behind the jaw and in front of the ear
- dry skin or rashes
- vaginal dryness
- a dry, persistent cough
- prolonged fatigue

The condition may cause damage to multiple systems and organs including the thyroid, kidneys, liver, lungs, nerves, and skin.

The specific cause of Sjogren's syndrome is unknown. A genetic connection is suspected, but a triggering mechanism, like a viral or bacterial infection, appears to be necessary.

Sarcoidosis

With sarcoidosis small collections of inflammatory cells form in the lungs, lymph nodes, eyes, and skin as well as other parts of the body.

The exact cause is not known, but the formations are believed to be in response to some inhaled substance. Most patients require only modest treatment protocols.

Sarcoidosis may be self-limiting, or progressively damage organs over a period of years.

Both the severity and speed of onset vary depending on the organs affected. Some patients are asymptomatic. These cases are diagnosed by accident when an X-ray is ordered for another reason. The major symptoms, if present include:

- fatigue
- fever
- swollen lymph nodes
- weight loss

Eventually, all sarcoidosis patients experience lung problems including:

- persistent dry cough
- wheezing
- chest pain
- shortness of breath

In 25% of cases skin problems also develop including:

- An inflamed and tender red / purple rash on the shins and ankles.
- Disfiguring skin sores on the cheeks, nose, and ears.
- Pigment changes that may be darker or lighter.
- Subcutaneous nodules around scars or tattoos.

Potential problems with the eyes and vision include:

- blurring
- pain
- severe redness
- sensitivity to light

Chronic sarcoidosis can cause the following long-term effects:

- Irreversible damage to the tissues between the air sacs in the lung affecting the ability to breathe.

- Severe eye inflammation progressing to eventual blindness and (more rarely) cataracts and glaucoma.

- Alterations in the body's ability to process calcium leading to kidney failure.

- Granulomas (granulated masses of tissue) in the heart that disrupt electrical signals and cause abnormal rhythms.

In a small number of sarcoidosis cases granulomas also form in the brain and spinal cord where they disrupt the activities of the central nervous system. Facial paralysis develops if the facial nerves become inflamed.

Lupus

In cases of lupus (systemic lupus erythematosus) the

body's immune system malfunctions, attacking and damaging various tissues. Symptoms include:

- deep fatigue
- persistent low-grade fever
- severe joint pain
- muscle aches
- skin rash (face or body)
- extreme sun sensitivity
- weight loss
- mental confusion
- seizures
- chest pain on taking a deep breath
- nose, mouth, or throat sores
- enlarged lymph nodes
- poor circulation in the extremities
- hair loss

Lupus cannot be cured. Patients can lead a normal but challenging life unless the function of major organs is threatened. Successful management relies on medication and associated care protocols.

Chiari Malformation

A Chiari malformation (CM) exists when the cerebellum sits too low in the rear of the skull, below the funnel-like opening for the spinal canal called the foramen magnum. The resulting pressure blocks the flow of cerebrospinal fluid (CSF), which surrounds and cushions both the brain and the spinal cord.

Developmental defects, genetic mutations, or poor prenatal nutrition cause primary or congenital CM. Injury, infection, or an exposure to harmful substances leads to excessive drainage of spinal fluid, which can cause secondary or acquired CM. Four classifications indicate severity and the parts of the brain protruding into the spinal canal:

- **Type 1**: The lower cerebellum (cerebellar tonsils) extends into the foramen magnum, but does not involve the brain stem. This is the most common CM and often causes no symptoms. Type 1 is first detected in adolescence or young adulthood during an examination for another condition and is the only acquired CM.

- **In Type II** or classic CM both cerebellar and brain stem tissue extends into the foramen magnum. The nerves connecting the two halves of the cerebellum, the cerebellar vermis are absent or incomplete. Myelomeningocele, a form of spina bifida, often accompanies Type II CM. The spinal canal and backbone fail to close before birth. The spinal cord and its protective membrane protrude through a sac-like opening in the back, with partial or complete paralysis occurring below this protrusion.

- **In Type III**, the most serious CM, the cerebellum and brain stem herniate through the foramen magnum and into the spinal cord causing severe neurological defects. The protrusion can include the brain's fourth ventricle, which connects to the upper parts of the brain and circulates CSF. In a small percentage of cases, the herniated tissue enters the pouch-like occipital encephalocele at the back of the head or neck or the covering of the brain and spinal cord protrude from an abnormal opening at the rear of the skull.

- In the rare **Type IV** CM, parts of the cerebellum are missing (cerebellar hypoplasia), and portions of the skull and spinal cord are visible even though the cerebellar tonsils are in their normal location.

CM symptoms include:

- neck pain
- balance problems
- dizziness
- muscular weakness
- abnormal sensation in the extremities
- visual problems
- difficulty swallowing
- ringing or buzzing in the ears
- hearing loss
- vomiting
- insomnia
- depression
- headache
- loss of hand / eye coordination
- deterioration of fine motor skills

In infants, expected symptoms include irritability at mealtime, difficulty swallowing, gagging, vomiting, excessive drooling, an inability to gain weight, a weak cry, a stiff neck, breathing problems, and developmental delays.

Deconditioning

When an organism adapts to a less demanding environment the decreased physical activity results in muscle loss called "deconditioning."

Illness, orthopedic casting, aging, paralysis, and low gravity environments (space exploration), all cause deconditioning. The abnormal distribution of bodily fluids under these circumstances, including blood volume changes, can trigger a POTS episode.

Delta Storage Pool Deficiency

A deficiency in dense granules in blood platelets causes Delta Storage Pool Deficiency, a condition discovered in the 1970s. Dense granules release chemicals necessary for clotting. The major symptoms include:

- bleeding in the nose and mouth
- bruising
- potential severe bleeding from injuries
- excessive menstrual bleeding
- bleeding complications in childbirth

To diagnose Delta SPD blood work is taken to measure clotting time and platelet aggregation (clumping). Microscopic studies reveal the number of dense granules and help doctors to eliminate other platelet disorders.

No medicine exists to increase the number of dense

granules. Medications used to maintain the condition include DDAVP to —improve clotting, and Amicar, which interrupts the breakdown of clots. Prior to surgery, patients with Delta SPD may require a platelet transfusion.

Patients should avoid aspirin and nonsteroidal anti-inflammatories like ibuprofen and naproxen and mitigate activities with an increased risk of bleeding.

Ehlers Danlos Syndrome

The inherited collagen protein disorders collectively named Ehlers Danlos Syndrome causes hyper-flexible joints. Concurrently, fragile, "stretchy" skin and veins may make wound stitching difficult or even impossible.

The more severe Vascular Ehlers-Danlos may lead to rupturing of blood vessels, the intestines, or the uterus. Patients with this variant of the syndrome should seek genetic counseling before starting a family.

Symptoms include:

- loose joints that move beyond a normal range
- weakened connective tissue that can be stretched beyond normal limits
- slowly healing skin with excessive scarring
- harmless fatty lumps around the knees or elbows

People with Vascular Ehlers-Danlos syndrome tend to exhibit distinctive facial features including a thin nose, thin upper lip, small earlobes and prominent eyes. The skin appears translucent and bruises easily. The underlying blood vessels may also be visible.

Mononucleosis

A virus transmitted through saliva causes infectious mononucleosis. Labeled the "kissing disease," mono can also be passed on through a cough or sneeze or by sharing eating utensils.

The disease is not as contagious as the common cold and is most prevalent and severe in adolescents and young adults. The virus incubates for 4-6 weeks before some combination of the following symptoms manifest:

- fatigue
- overall malaise
- sore throat
- fever
- swollen lymph nodes (neck and armpits)
- swollen tonsils
- headache
- skin rash
- soft, swollen spleen

The fever and sore throat diminish after 2 weeks, but the fatigue, enlarged lymph nodes, and swollen spleen take an additional 2 weeks or more to resolve. Rest and good hydration are essential for recovery.

Epstein Barr Virus

The Epstein–Barr virus (EBV) causes infectious mononucleosis, and is associated with Hodgkin's lymphoma, Burkitt's lymphoma, nasopharyngeal carcinoma, and conditions appearing with HIV.

Researchers believe infection with Epstein-Barr elevates the risk for the development of other autoimmune diseases including dermatomyositis (an inflammatory connective tissue disease), systemic lupus erythematosus, rheumatoid arthritis, Sjögren's syndrome, and multiple sclerosis.

The virus, which is part of the herpes family, is transmitted through saliva and also via genital secretions.

Lyme Disease

Deer ticks in North America and Europe spread Lyme disease, caused by the bacterium *Borrelia burgdorferi.* People who spend time in wooded or grassy areas face the greatest risk. Patients who receive appropriate antibiotics quickly recover completely, but later stage treatment progresses more slowly.

Early signs and symptoms (within one month of infection) include:

- A small, inflamed bump at the site of the tick bite that expands into a bull's eye pattern called an erythema migrans rash.

- Fever, chills, headache, and body aches.

Later stage symptoms include:

- Severe joint pain and swelling, especially in the knees.

- Meningitis (inflammation of the membranes surrounding the brain.)

- Bell's Palsy (temporary paralysis of one side of the face.)

- Weakness and numbness in the limbs with impaired muscle movement.

Less common symptoms include:

- Irregular heartbeat.
- Eye inflammation.
- Liver inflammation.
- Debilitating fatigue.

Untreated Lyme disease can spread throughout the body for years after the initial infection and contribute to neurological problems and the development of arthritis.

Extra-Pulmonary Mycoplasma Pneumonia

The bacteria species *Mycoplasma pneumoniae,* spread through respiratory droplet transmission, causes mycoplasma or "walking" pneumonia.

Unlike other forms of pneumonia, this protracted illness causes pharyngitis and bronchitis. The protracted course of walking pneumonia, which can become chronic, may play a role in the development of rheumatoid arthritis and other rheumatological diseases.

Hepatitis C

The chronic liver infection Hepatitis C, though often asymptomatic, causes scarring and ultimately cirrhosis. Liver failure, cancer, and life-threatening esophageal and gastric varices (enlarged veins) may result. Primary blood-to-blood transmission may be from intravenous drug use, blood transfusions, or poorly sterilized medical equipment.

Treatment in 50-80% of cases results in a cure, but Hepatitis C remains the leading cause of liver transplantations. Standard drugs used to combat the disease include peginterferon, ribavirin, boceprevir and telaprevir. There is no vaccine against Hepatitis C.

Multiple Sclerosis

The inflammatory disease multiple sclerosis (MS) damages the insulating covers of nerve cells in the brain and spinal cord disrupting the communication network of the central nervous system. MS can follow a relapsing, remitting course. Patients suffer isolated attacks or progressively worsening symptoms that over time lead to permanent neurological damage.

Researchers do not know the exact cause of MS, but genetic

and environmental factors are believed to play a role. There is no cure. Treatment focuses on improving function following an attack and preventing future episodes. The disease appears twice as often in women with onset between the ages of 20 and 50.

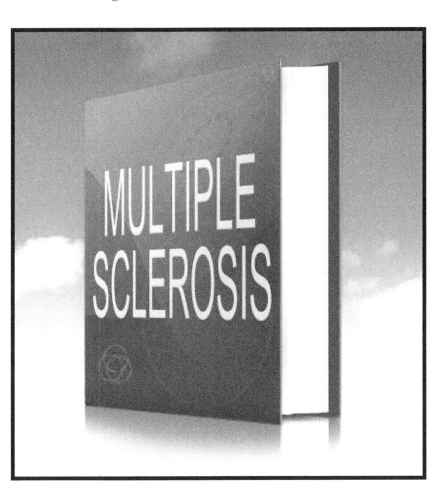

Other Conditions

Other conditions or circumstances that may include POTS symptoms include:

- mitochondrial disorders (blood cell defects)
- mast cell activation disorders (histamine and inflammatory reactions)
- paraneoplastic syndrome (a rare immune system response)
- alcoholism
- chemotherapy
- heavy metal poisoning
- pregnancy
- surgery
- trauma
- vaccinations
- vitamin deficiencies
- anemia

Part 2 - Signs and Symptoms

POTS cannot be reduced to a simple description like, "I stand up and then I faint." There are numerous signs and symptoms associated with the syndrome.

When some combination of the following has been in place for six months or more and the correct tests have been performed, a definitive diagnosis is more likely.

- A feeling of being lightheaded upon standing with possible heart palpitations and a "tremulous" or shaky feeling.

- Some type of visual disturbance like "seeing stars" or blurring.

- An uncomfortable feeling in the head (throbbing) and possibly in the neck.

- An inability to concentrate or think clearly. Often described as "brain fog."

- Feeling tired and experiencing weakness.

- Fainting spells, generally within 10 minutes of standing.

- Nausea or "queasiness."

- Discomfort in the chest including being short of breath.

POTS patients often experience difficulty with associated anxiety as they become increasingly apprehensive about standing. This leads to additional symptoms including:

- Gastrointestinal upsets like constipation and bloating and/or episodes of diarrhea.

- Changes in sweating, usually increased with a sense of feeling "clammy."

- Insomnia that exacerbates the overall problem of fatigue.

In cases with POTS-like symptoms, any or all of the following diagnostic tests may be used to arrive at an explanation for what is happening to the body, particularly within the autonomic nervous system.

Diagnostic Testing

Each of the following 10 diagnostic tests is routinely used to evaluate patients suffering from symptoms typically seen in POTS. All are designed to understand aspects of blood flow and nerve function as they relate to posture and other external stimuli.

Multiple tests are employed in an effort to create a complete picture of exactly what precedes an episode.

Posture Study

The posture study monitors heart rate, blood pressure, and

the plasma concentrations that regulate them when the patient is lying down and standing. Blood is drawn from an IV in the arm during the test. The patient lies still while baseline readings are taken. The patient then stands up for 30 minutes while the measurements are repeated.

POTS patients will show an increased heart rate of 30 beats per minute when they stand and an accompanying drop in blood pressure of < 20/10 mm Hg. Some will also show elevated norepinephrine levels of > 600pg/mL.

Head Up Tilt Table

Doctors use the tilt table to evaluate cardiovascular response to positional changes. In POTS cases they are looking for a sudden drop in blood pressure with either an increase in pulse rate or fainting when the patient is upright.

To perform the test, the patient lies on the table with straps around the abdomen and legs and then is gradually tilted upright between 60-80 degrees for 45 minutes. The intended purpose is to replicate the patient's problem in a controlled setting.

POTS patients will show an increase in heart rate of > 30 beats/minute during the head up tilt with little or no change in blood pressure, usually < 20/10 mm Hg.

Cardiac Output

A cardiac output test judges the amount of blood the heart

can pump by measuring pulmonary blood flow. The patient is forced to breathe through the mouth while wearing a device containing oxygen and two inert gases. A clamp renders respiration through the nose impossible.

One of the inert gases is blood soluble, disappearing as the patient breathes in direct proportion to the rate of pulmonary blood flow. The other gas does not enter the bloodstream, therefore allowing for lung volume to also be measured.

(Note that there are other methods for measuring cardiac output. This method is, however, quite common.)

Beat-to-Beat Blood Pressure

Beat-to-beat blood pressure testing non-invasively tracks changes in response to various tests through a bracelet-like wrist device with a Velcro strap secured around one finger. This monitor is worn for the duration of any other type of testing being performed.

Valsalva Maneuver

In the Valsalva maneuver, the patient blows against a resisting surface for several seconds followed by a period of relaxation. The action of the blowing increases pressure in the chest and abdomen, forcing blood out of the chest and down into the arms with a brief increase in blood pressure. This is referred to as Phase I.

The stroke volume, which is the amount of blood ejected by

the heart with each beat, plummets due to the decreased entry of blood from the veins as a consequence of the straining. The brain senses these changes as well as the concurrent increases in nerve traffic causing more norepinephrine to be released. This tightens blood vessels throughout the body. This is Phase II.

Phase III begins when the patient relaxes, causing a brief drop in blood pressure before the blood rushes back into the chest. Blood pressure increases in Phase IV and since the blood vessels are constricted, an overshoot of blood pressure is produced, outflow falls, and with it the heart rate.

Observing these various changes and their rate and interaction gives physicians information about sympathetic and parasympathetic function. Patients with the kind of autonomic dysfunction present in POTS will likely have an exaggerated blood pressure increases in Phases II and IV.

Sinus Arrhythmia

Heart rate normally varies with the breath, increasing when we breathe in and decreasing when we breathe out. These changes, which are controlled by the parasympathetic nervous systems are called respiratory sinus arrhythmia.

In a sinus arrhythmia test, the patient's heart rate is monitored while taking a series of deep breaths, roughly six per minute. A difference of 15 beats between minimum and maximum heart rate is considered within normal range.

Typically patients with POTS will have normal results on this test, but if abnormalities do show up, they may suggest a diagnosis of a condition other than POTS or of a condition present in conjunction with POTS.

Transcranial Doppler

A Transcranial Doppler test determines the velocity of cerebral blood flow. The patient is in an upright position, standing or on a tilt board. A Doppler probe placed near the temple emits high-frequency sound waves that are used to map the speed of blood flow in the cerebral vessels. In patients with POTS the expected results would be decreased velocity when in an upright position.

Cold Pressor Test

During a cold pressor test the patient plunges their hand in a tub of ice cold water and leaves it submerged for 1-2 minutes while both heart rate and blood pressure are monitored.

The normal reflexive action is an increase in heart rate and systolic blood pressure. A patient with POTS, however, will show increases in systolic and diastolic blood pressure much greater than those observed in normal individuals.

QSART Testing

The QSART is a sweat test that gauges the ability of sympathetic nerves in the skin to release acetylcholine. If the individual has lost sympathetic nerve terminals, no sweat will be produced. If the person has a brain abnormality that inhibits sweat production as the temperature increases, they will still sweat during a QSART test. Therefore, the QSART helps to distinguish between loss of terminals and misregulation of signals sent along the sympathetic nerves.

The test is performed by wiping the leg and wrist with acetone and then alcohol. This cleans and dries the skin. Next, four electrodes are placed on three areas of the leg and one of the wrist.

The electrodes are filled with acetylcholine, which is activated with a mild electrical current to stimulate sweat gland activity while allowing the body to release its own acetylcholine causing sweating in adjacent sites. The entire procedure requires about 45 minutes.

Measuring the degree of sweating response helps doctors to determine the exact nature of sympathetic dysfunction that may be contributing to the symptoms seen in POTS.

Endothelial Function

The Endothelial Function test judges the function of the cells that line the blood vessels. A baseline blood pressure reading is taken first before an uninflated blood pressure cuff is placed on the non-dominant arm for later use. The index finger of each hand is then placed inside a plastic cylinder called an EndoPat probe, which will measure arterial tone.

Baseline readings are again taken while the patient sits still for 5 minutes, at which time the blood pressure cuff is inflated to a level greater than the systolic blood pressure for the purpose of stopping blood flow for 5 minutes. Then the cuff is deflated and additional readings taken over another 5 minute period.

Part 3 - Causes and Treatment

Now we know the specific symptoms of POTS, the groups most at risk, and what diagnostic tools doctors use in these cases. If you or your loved one suffers from POTS, these general descriptions don't delve deeply enough into the mechanics of the underlying dysfunction to help you interpret the information you are likely receiving.

Regardless of the specific cause or associated conditions, POTS stems directly from a malfunction of the autonomic nervous system. The term "nervous system," while used colloquially to imply one uniform network of nerves, does not do justice to the complexity of the body's neural control structure.

The Autonomic Nervous System

The human nervous system interprets information derived from the senses and sends orders to the muscles and glands. Nerves control function we don't have to think about, like digestion and circulation, and are also responsible for both thoughts and moods.

The brain and spinal cord comprise the central nervous system, while all the nerves that branch outward from these structures form the peripheral nervous system.

Nerves that regulate the movement of skeletal muscles are described as "somatic," while those that regulate involuntary functions including heart rate and digestion are termed "autonomic."

There are two divisions of the autonomic nervous system, sympathetic and parasympathetic.

- The sympathetic nerves control "fight or flight" reactions by increasing heart rate, constricting blood flow in the peripheral arteries, and raising blood pressure.

- The parasympathetic nerves work while the body is at rest and under normal conditions. They decrease heart rate and stimulate digestion.

It may be easier to think of the two symptoms as complete opposites. The sympathetic nervous system deals with action or stimulation, while the parasympathetic handles rest or tranquil functions.

Dysautonomia

POTS is a form of dysautonomia, a blanket term covering any neuropathy (nerve dysfunction) affecting the autonomic nerves. In the case of POTS, a change in posture triggers the malfunction.

There are many forms of dysautonomia, for instance:

- **Autonomic Dysreflexia (AD)** - In individuals with a spinal cord injury the nerves below the injury misinterpret signals from an irritation and cause flushing, a spike in blood pressure, and nasal stuffiness. If not treated, AD can lead to a stroke.

- **Diabetic Autonomic Neuropathy** - Diabetic Autonomic Neuropathy is the most common form of dysautonomia globally, affecting 69 million people. The conditions causes tingling and a "pins and needles" sensation in the extremities and indicates an elevated risk for a cardiovascular event.

- **Reflex Sympathetic Dystrophy** - Reflex Sympathetic Dystrophy or Complex Regional Pain Syndrome causes chronic pain most often in an arm or leg. The exact trigger is unknown, but the resulting inflammation and swelling in the affected limb are tied to nerve damage.

As we have seen, multiple conditions can cause the orthostatic intolerance that is the hallmark of POTS, but regardless of the precipitating event, the results are a form of dysautonomia.

Effects of Posture on Blood Flow

Under normal circumstances when we lie down, a quarter of our blood supply resides in the chest cavity. When we stand up, gravity draws 800 milliliters of blood down into the abdomen and into the legs.

The sympathetic nervous system immediately reacts to this gravitational pull by narrowing the blood vessels to maintain the correct blood supply to the brain. At the time same, our heart rate goes up about 10-15 beats per minute and there is a slight increase in blood pressure.

This system goes completely awry with someone who has POTS. The blood vessels become overly dilated so that blood puddles in the lower part of the body. Blood flow to the brain drops 20-30% and the heart races, shooting up 30-40 beats per minute.

Specific POTS Case: Patrick's Story

In an October 17, 2011 article for *The New York Times*, "Ailment Can Steal Youth from the Young," Jane E. Brody describes the case of then 14-year-old Patrick Fox.

Over the course of a year a cavalcade of doctors worked with the boy — pediatricians, cardiologists, rheumatologists, and even a geneticist. None could explain his fatigue, racing heart, aching body, headaches, or tendency to overheat.

When Patrick could hardly leave his bed, the doctors began to say he was a lazy, depressed, manipulative child who should see a psychiatrist, in spite of his history of being an active young man who enjoyed school and did well in his studies.

When his mother finally took him to the Mayo Clinic after the boy experienced chest pains, they received a diagnosis within two hours — POTS. With proper supporting treatment, Patrick returned to his classes and took up sports again, rapidly regaining his status as an honors student.

Dr. Julian M. Stewart, a researcher at Westchester Medical Center and New York Medical College quoted in the article said, "These people can't remain upright . . . [the] drop in cerebral flow when they try to stand up . . . causes cognitive difficulties; they can't think well on their feet."

Many teenage POTS patients like Patrick experience their first symptoms with a sudden growth spurt. In Patrick's case, he rapidly grew to 6' 2". After coming down with what seemed like the flu, the persistent symptoms settled in and grew more severe over time.

After the Mayo Clinic doctors put a name to the condition, Patrick followed the guidelines they suggested and sought acupuncture treatments in an effort to normalize his heart rate.

(Although there have been no controlled clinical trials of the use of acupuncture with POTS, many patients like Patrick say the supportive therapy helped. If you are interested in this topic see "Acupuncture Effect and Central Autonomic Regulation, by Qian-Qian Li, Guang-Xia Shi, Qian Xu, Jing Wang, Cun-Zhi Liu,* and Lin-Peng Wang in Evid Based Complement Alternat Med. 2013; 2013: 267959. Published online May 26, 2013. The paper is online at www.ncbi.nlm.nih.gov/pmc/articles/PMC3677642/.)

In developmental cases like Patrick's, a fairly standard protocol is used to manage the POTS symptoms until they abate on their own with growth.

Standard Treatments and Lifestyle Changes

The standard approach to treating developmental POTS

symptoms focuses on increasing blood volume and building both strength and energy. The treatments and lifestyle changes recommended by the Mayo Clinic include the following.

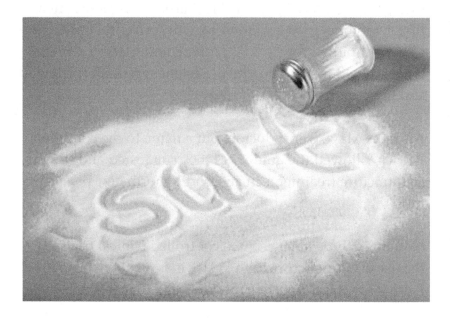

High Salt Diet

The average American consumes 3,436 mg of salt per day. Under normal circumstances, that consumption is appallingly high. The recommended intake for healthy blood pressure and heart function is 1,500 mg even though the human body only needs 180-500 mg.

POTS patients, however, should consume 5,000 mg of salt per day and in some cases, as much as 10,000 mg. Clearly this would be dangerous for older patients with high blood pressure, cardiovascular, or kidney disease. Such an eating program should only be attempted with strict medical supervision, and is not applicable to all forms of POTS.

Some palatable ways of increasing salt intake include:

- salt watermelon or avocado wedges
- mix extra salt in peanut butter to taste
- use beef jerky or salami as a snack
- eat more scrambled eggs, which hide the taste of salt
- drink bouillon, V8, tomato, or pickle juice
- use soy sauce as a condiment

Clearly you don't want to completely sacrifice good nutrition, but according to WebMD, Heart.org, and similar sites, the foods with the highest concentration of sodium include:

- frozen dinners
- ready-to-eat cereals
- vegetable juices
- packaged deli meats
- processed cheese
- salad dressings
- canned soups
- canned vegetable
- tomato sauce
- salty peanuts
- pizza
- blended coffee drinks

This is one case where you must read labels in reverse and avoid products that are "heart healthy" or "low sodium."

The goal of increasing salt intake is to increase both blood pressure and the circulatory volume of the blood itself. Blood with a high salt content holds more water.

Fluid Intake

With the recommended high salt intake, staying well hydrated is essential. POTS patients should, at minimum, drink 3-4 liters of fluids each day. These should be non-caffeinated beverages like water, milk, juices, soups, and sports drinks.

As an indicator that fluid consumption has reached or exceeded the recommended level, the patient's urine should be completely clear.

Sleep

Rather than give in to the constant need to nap, POTS patients should stay as active as possible during regular day-to-day activities, but commit to a regular schedule of 9 hours of sleep per night.

For people who have difficulty falling asleep, a set routine is essential. Go to bed at the same time each night and get up at the same time the next day.

Avoid stimulants for 2 or 3 hours before bedtime, including not just food and drink but also vigorous exercise or any kind of exceptionally engaging mental activity. Try dimming the lights in the room and listening to environmental sounds or soothing music.

Medications

Drugs are not always used to treat POTS, but some medications can be useful in addressing symptoms. These include beta blockers to lower heart rate, and midodrine to constrict outlying blood vessels.

Other drugs used include fludrocortisone to increase salt retention and blood volume, and antidepressant to raise serotonin levels in the brain.*

(Note that the use of selective serotonin reuptake inhibitors or SSRIs with POTS is controversial. Some doctors say this class of anti-depressant is helpful, while others say the drugs have no efficacy whatsoever.)

Exercises for Autonomic Disorders

Exercise is a recommended component of treatment for any autonomic disorder including POTS. Your doctor or physical therapist will assign goals and stipulate target heart ranges to achieve but not exceed.

If you are exercising at home, you will likely need a "workout buddy" so you are not alone if you experience any negative symptoms. This is especially important if you'll be at a local gym. A knowledgeable personal trainer or physical therapist is invaluable to your progress, and many hospitals maintain rehabilitation facilities that employ such people.

Such a setting also allows for vital signs to be monitored

during your workout, data that is valuable to your physician in assessing your progress. In cases of severe deconditioning, a brief stay in an in-patient physical therapy program is an option as well.

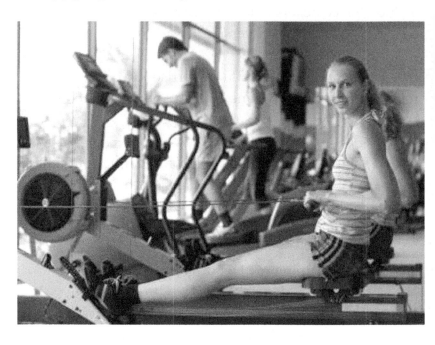

Unless your physical therapist or personal trainer understands POTS, you could be assigned inappropriate upright exercises like walking on a treadmill or riding an upright exercise bike.

The best exercises are those that cause no orthostatic stress. Reclined stretches, yoga positions, and weight lifting as well as seated exercises on recumbent bikes or rowing machines are good choices, as is swimming.

The patient must build up tolerance over time and should not attempt upright exercises for several months. (Note that this varies from case to case.)

Dysautonomia International provides the following home exercises tips. REMEMBER, never start an exercise program without consulting your doctor!

Beginning Gentle Movements

Remember to be patient with yourself, especially if you are suffering from reconditioning as a consequence of a long period of inactivity. Remember that even 1-2 minutes a day is progress, so long as you stay with it and work to increase your tolerance.

- **Leg Pillow Squeeze** - In a reclining position, place a folded pillow between your needs. Squeeze and hold for 10 seconds. Repeat.

- **Arm Pillow Squeeze** - Fold the pillow and squeeze it between your hands in a "praying" position for 10 seconds. Repeat.

- **Alphabet Toes** - In a reclining position, lift your leg slightly and write your name in the air with your toes. Build toward doing the whole alphabet several times a day.

- **Side Leg Lifts** - Lie on your side and lift your leg up and then down without touching your legs together. Repeat.

- **Front Leg Lifts** - Lying on your back, lift your leg until your toe is pointed at the ceiling. Repeat and then switch to the other leg.

Remember that any kind of stretching will help your blood to move around your body and will take stress off of your joints. Go through your whole body simply performing mild stretches with your feet, legs, back, arms, and neck. Going through this sequence when you wake up in the morning is a great way to start the day. Use the same technique to help relax before going to sleep at night.

Recumbent Cardio

Many patients will be able to begin at this level if they have not experienced a long period of deconditioning. Plan on stretching 5-10 minutes to warm up before doing the exercises.

Discuss a target heart rate with your doctor. Most patients can tolerate 75-80% of their maximum heart rate, but this can be affected by currently prescribed medications.

Purchasing a heart rate monitor is a good idea to more accurately work within your set target range. The most accurate units are the ones that place the sensor on the chest where it is held in place with a strap. Finger-based units are not as accurate for patients experiencing problems with peripheral blood flow.

- **Rowing** - For indoors a rowing machine is excellent, but if possible, plan on graduating to using a kayak or similar boat outdoors. Start slowly, going 2-5 minutes per day. Work toward 45 minutes per day, 5 days a week, with 30 minutes performed within the target heart rate zone.

- **Recumbent Biking** - Recumbent exercise bikes allow riders to pedal in a seated position. As with rowing, begin with just a few minutes per day, working up to 45 minutes a day, five days a week, with 30 minutes at the target heart rate.

- **Swimming** - The pressure of being in the water helps to prevent orthostatic symptoms so even those patients with forms of dysautonomia that have kept them bedridden for years are able to stand upright in a pool for as much as an hour. Begin by stretching and strength training in the water with an exercise "buddy" and work toward actual swimming sessions. It's possible to get a well-rounded cardio routine in the water that will tone your legs and build the muscles of your core.

- **Weight Training** - Weight training is extremely useful to increase muscle tone and strength, which in turn leads the body to use oxygen more efficiently. Place particular emphasis on the leg and core muscles. Begin with weight machines that allow you to work in a reclined or seated position Be cautious about lifting your arms over your head.

Normal Workouts

Achieving a level of conditioning that allows for 45 minutes of exercise (including cardio) for at least 3 days a week with emphasis on leg and core strength is an excellent goal. Some patients recover so well that they are able to jog, run, or walk several miles per week.

Again, do not attempt an exercise program without first consulting with your doctor. If your POTS symptoms occur in concert with other conditions like:

- **Ehlers Danlos Syndrome** – One of several inherited collagen protein disorders discussed earlier in this text.

- **Joint Hypermobility Syndrome** - A benign syndrome that often exists in concert with POTS in which the patient's joints move beyond the normally expected range of motion.

- **Mitochondrial Disease** – Disease that results from the failure of specialized compartments in the body's blood cells called the mitochondria.

- **Hyperkalemic Periodic Paralysis** – A disorder characterized by periodic episodes of muscular weakness and also higher than normal levels of blood potassium.

- **electrolyte imbalances** – Electrolytes are chemicals in the blood that regulate numerous important bodily functions. Imbalances can results from loss of bodily fluids from vomiting, diarrhea, sweating, or a high fever, or from dietary or hormonal issues, kidney disease, or as a consequence of chemotherapy.

- **diabetes** – A disease affecting the body's production and processing of glucose. Discussed earlier in this text.

- **Myasthenia Gravis** – Also known as Lou Gehrig's Disease, this condition causes an abnormal and irreversible weakening and atrophy of the muscles. Autoimmune in nature.

- **heart problems** – This can be any one of a number of cardiovascular problems, especially those affecting circulation, heart rate, and blood pressure.

- **or asthma (among others)** . . . – Asthma is a respiratory condition involving spasms of the bronchi in the lungs causing severe breathing difficulties.

there are special considerations that must be met for a safe and successful fitness routine.

Specific POTS Case: With an Underlying Cause

There are many people living with POTS who blog about their experiences or discuss their illness and symptoms in forums online. At POTSgrrl, "a blog about Postural Orthostatic Tachycardia Syndrome for tweens, teens and everyone else interested in POTS," the author includes a post entitled "How to Find a POTS Doctor."

(See: potsgrrl.blogspot.com/p/doctorsmedical-centers-that-can.html.)

The story describes her odyssey in arriving at a diagnosis:

"It took me 9 months to get a diagnosis and that is actually pretty fast compared to other people. I went to over 30 different specialists, I had dozens of Emergency Room visits, and I ended up being admitted to the hospital three different times, to five different hospitals (for a total of 3 months in the hospital in one year) and NO ONE, not even the big shot neurologists, cardiologists and medical school professors I consulted with could figure me out. I misdiagnosed with all sorts of ridiculous diseases - neuroendocrine cancer, croup, bronchitis, pleurisy, panic attacks, etc. I didn't have any of those things. Seriously, when is the last time bronchitis caused someone to lose 60 lbs. and pass out every day for months on end?"

In the end, the author did her own research and presented journal articles from the Mayo Clinic to her neurologist, asking if she could have POTS. The doctor admitted he knew little about the condition, but agreed to read the materials and then consulted experts in the field. Based on those exchanges, a diagnosis was made.

This led to an equally long search for physicians specializing in autonomic disorders. In the end, the author finally found help at the Cleveland Clinic in Ohio where it was discovered that the underlying cause for the POTS was

Sjorgren's Syndrome.

Specific POTS Case: Jodi Epstein Rhum, Activist

Jodi Epstein Rhum grew up with an undiagnosed though mild case of POTS. Two of her four children have POTS and one suffers from Ehlers-Danlos Syndrome.

The former middle school teacher became an advocate for POTS awareness and is an active public speaker and author. She is Vice President of the Board of Directors of Dysautonomia International.

In 2011, she coauthored *POTS – Together We Stand: Riding the Waves of Dysautonomia* with Svetlana Blishteyn, which is an invaluable account of life with POTS by someone who has experienced it both as a patient and a mother.

(Please note, however, that this is a memoir and not a "living with" sort of guide.)

Rhum also maintains a presence on Facebook at: www.facebook.com/jodi.epsteinrhum

POTS Bloggers

At the time of this writing (mid-2014) the following blogs discussing life with POTS were all active. Like all things online, I cannot guarantee how long they will remain so, but I do believe that reading first-hand experiences with the syndrome and with the medical community is a crucial component of understanding and overcoming this condition, regardless of its underlying cause.

I am including an excerpt from each blog's description or "About Me" section following the title as an indicator of tone and content – and also because they offer further snapshots into the effects POTS can have on a person's life.

Please be aware that a blog is a personal online journal and many express extreme frustrations regarding long-term illness. Be forewarned that the modes of expression may be direct and at times profane.

Miss POTS – "Miss" as in Misdiagnosed
misspots.blogspot.com

"Miss POTS is my secret blog. It's where I can come and vent and curse and cry and find answers why . . . why do I have POTS? How can I fix this s**t? When ill it end?"

Musings of a Dysautonomiac
dysautonomiac.com

"Hello, and welcome! I was diagnosed with postural orthostatic tachycardia syndrome (POTS) in February, 2011, after years of symptoms. Having POTS has added many challenges to my life, and there are still days where I miss the life I used to have. But, I'm doing what I can to live my life in spite of POTS. I decided to create this blog to share with family and friends the difficulties of suffering from a chronic illness and to connect with other dysautonomia sufferers around the globe."

My Zebra Soup – Life with Dysautonomia
zebrasoup.me

"Life with Dysautonomia (POTS & NCS/NMH), MCAD, Ehlers Danlos Syndrome III, Small Fiber Neuropathy, Erythromelalgia, RLS, multiple disorders of the spine, ASD, Visual Snow, Hemiplegic Migraine, MTHFR & other comorbid conditions on my own terms. These hoofbeats definitely belong to a ZEBRA! "

Overcoming: Life with a Chronic Illness
hopealways.wordpress.com

"Hi. I'm a writer, musician, big dreamer, deep thinker, science nerd, and … a Dysautonomiapatient.
My life was very busy and active until I was diagnosed with this chronic, incurable illness. BUT, I AM DETERMINED TO GET BETTER. Here, I will be blogging about my life with a chronic illness – symptoms, experiences, advice, positivity, and encouragement in hopes of inspiring other people who struggle with chronic diseases."

POTS & OI Recovery
www.potsrecovery.com

"The author of this blog (me) has a condition called Postural Orthostatic Tachycardia Syndrome and Orthostatic Intolerance. Both conditions fall under the category of Dysautonomia: problems with the body's autonomic system. The conditions are not particulalry well known in the medical community and can be left undiagnosed in patients for years."

Stop POTS (and Dysautonomia!)
stoppotsvirginia.blogspot.com

"As of January 2012, I am a mother of 2 and a wife of 1. My son is almost 4, and my new daughter is 4 months old. Right now they are my world, along with my husband, because I am homebound - and often bedbound- due to POTS and a slew of other fun medical issues. My educational background and passion is marine biology. I worked in a number of research labs while at my University, co-authored and wrote for scientific journal publication, and as a paid scuba diver in the Keys during a stint in graduate school with every intention of getting my doctoral degree before having to leave mid semester when I first started having tachycardia and dizzy flares (in 2002/2003.)

(Please note that the author indicated in a special note that updates on this site were discontinued in 2013.)

Teens with POTS: Living with Dysautonomia
teenswithpots.wordpress.com
"My name is Jenna and I am a Freshman in college living with a chronic illness. I blog to release my frustrations, to share my happiness, and to connect with others who are in similar predicaments. My goal in my writing is for someone somewhere to feel like they're not alone. Happy reading! "

With a Side of Salt: POTS Support

withasideofsaltpotssupport.blogspot.com

"My name is Crista Procopio and I am a POTS patient at the Mayo Clinic. I have lived with POTS my entire life but I unfortunately went undiagnosed until a few years ago. Please feel free to read my story below. "

(See the About Me link for a complete story of Procopio's diagnosis and life with POTS.)

P.O.T.S Become Aware

potsbecomeaware.blogspot.com

"This blog is to raise awareness of Postural Orthostatic Tachycardia Syndrome. I hope to be able to help others that are dealing with the same things I am going through. Hopefully through this you will gain new insight, information, and support to know you are not alone in this struggle!"

(Please note that this blog has not been updated since 2011, but does contain an extensive first-person account under the "My Story" tab.)

Living with Bob (Dysautonomia)

bobisdysautonomia.blogspot.com

"*Living with Bob* is about finding the funny when faced with the absurd and disheartening world of chronic illness. It doesn't take life too seriously, instead choosing to face the crapfest that is my health with a large dose of black humour. There may be the occasional piece of useful medical information."

Dysautonomia Normal

michele-dysautonomianormal.blogspot.com

"I was normal until I was diagnosed with dysautonomia . . . dysautonomia is when your autonomic nervous system malfunctions. The autonomic nervous system controls things you don't think about like heart rate, digestion, respiration, perspiration, and pupil dilation to name a few. Anything you don't think about your body automatically does."

(Please note that this website has not been updated since February 2013.)

Cranberry Tea Time

www.cranberryteatime.com

"Hello, Friend, and welcome to Cranberry Tea Time! Thank you for coming to visit with me. I'm Rachel, a pastor's wife, a mother, and a sinner saved by grace. I like coffee, flowers, tea parties, the color purple, and painted toenails. I have never reached my chocolate threshold seriously think I may not have one. I have dysautonomia; it's an invisible illness, and it makes life challenging. I am learning to take life one day at a time, to rely on God's strength, and to rest in His grace. Despite the difficulties I face, I am very blessed. God has given me a wonderful family and blessings beyond what I deserve."

Part 4 - Living with POTS

POTS may be episodic and self-limiting or chronic. Young children tend to grow out of the symptoms, but in adults, major lifestyle and workplace accommodations may be necessary. In either case, it is imperative that the patients and the people advocating on their behalf know how to talk to "authorities" involved.

The following material on school system and workplace accommodations relates primarily to laws in the United States because that is the area with which I am most familiar.

Although the legal specifics may not apply to your case, the discussion should offer insight into what might be necessary to help a child or adult with POTS remain functional, productive and involved. Be sure to look for legislation protecting the disabled in your own country to find out your rights under the law.

Working with School Systems

In the United States, Section 504 of the Rehabilitation Act of 1973 requires that school districts make appropriate modifications for children with disabilities. Children with POTS often qualify for a "504 plan" that designs specific accommodations so they may continue successfully with their education.

(Educators can learn more on the Dysautonomia International site at www.dysautonomiainternational.org.

Click on the menu item for "Educators" for available resources including printable brochures that explain the basics of dysautonomic disorders.)

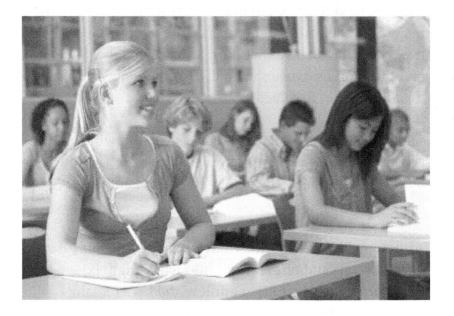

Since collaboration between educators and parents creates the most successful execution of this kind of planning, the following are some points to consider in arranging appropriate compensatory measures:

Symptom Management

As with any illness, students with POTS must manage their symptoms throughout the day with the help of their teachers and administrators. Provisions must be made for:

- Access to hydrating fluids throughout the day. The slightest degree of dehydration will make symptoms much worse. Students should be allowed to have their water bottles at all times.

- Salty snacks are essential for fluid retention, which in turn supports both blood volume and increased blood pressure. Like fluids, salt intake throughout the day is imperative.

- POTS students may have gastrointestinal upsets and, due to their high fluid requirement, will need many bathroom breaks for urination. The child should have a permanent bathroom pass to avoid being embarrassed in front of peers.

- Any activity that involves standing in line should be avoided or the child should be allowed to sit or to lie down. The longer a child with POTS remains upright, the greater the chance of blood pooling in the lower body. This can lead to dizziness, fatigue, nausea, and chest pain among other symptoms.

- Alternate sitting positions may be needed to avoid blood pooling. This may include elevating the feet, sitting on the knees, bringing the knees to the chest, or sitting cross legged. All help to regulate blood flow to the heart and should not be treated as disrespectful or "lazy" behavior. Flexing of the legs, stretching, and brief walks will also be needed.

Coping with Hypersensitivies

Children with POTS are sensitive to temperature and cannot always control their body temperature. For many, air conditioning and portable fans are a must. In school settings where a uniform is required, make sure the student is allowed to dress in layers that can be removed or added as needed.

Hypersensitivity to odors may cause headaches or vomiting, especially in science labs and art classrooms. Such areas should be well ventilated or the student should be allowed to wear some type of breathing protection. Ideally personnel and other students will be asked not to wear any perfume or use any personal care product that is strong or heavily scented.

Some POTS patients are sensitive to noise, light and vibration and must rely on sunglasses or earplugs in certain situations. These students may not be able to sit near a window or will require dim lighting.

Scheduling Considerations

POTS will lead to frequent, unpredictable absences for which the student should not be penalized.

Prioritize the day to emphasize core academics. Remember that the child will have limited energy that may not last for an entire school day.

Half days often work best. Many children with POTS often experience more severe symptoms in the morning when blood pressure is at its lowest. An early afternoon schedule may be more effective.

Academic Considerations

For partially homebound students, make sure teachers coordinate homework to avoid excessive workloads.

Consider engaging a tutor to help students facing extended absences. Have this person coordinate with the school to ensure work criteria are fulfilled.

Ask for a second set of books to keep at home. Managing severe fatigue is one of the great challenges with POTS. Carrying a heavy book bag wastes valuable energy.

Request that scheduled classes be as close together as possible to minimize the degree of walking during the day. The child should also be allowed extra time to make class changes. In cases of severe brain fog, students may not be able to remember a locker combination and may need a different means to secure their belongings.

In very large facilities some form of transportation like a wheelchair may be necessary to make successful class changes. If stairs are required, someone must walk with the child. Elevators should always be used when available.

Academic Performance

All teachers should be informed about the significance of brain fog (cerebral hypoperfusion) that exists with POTS. Patients grapple with decreased powers of concentration, memory storage and information retrieval.

Extended test time and frequent breaks will help exam scores. Altered testing times should be considered to accommodate stamina and attention span. If necessary, a quiet room should be offered to the student to aid with concentration.

If note taking is problematic, the child should be allowed to use a tape recorder or laptop and/or to have a "buddy" for note sharing. As math requires sequencing and multiple steps that may be difficult, get permission for the child to use a calculator.

Physical Education

Physical education classes should be modified or eliminated. Students with POTS cannot tolerate activities that require walking, running, standing, and involve rapid changes in posture.

Acceptable exercises are those that can be performed while lying down or in a seated position. Recumbent biking, rowing machines, and even swimming are all appropriate.

Drills and Emergencies

A special plan will be required for emergency situations and evacuations. The child should be assigned an adult "buddy" and relocated away from the alarm for any kind of drill since the noise may exacerbate existing symptoms.

The student should be allowed to carry a cell phone at all times in case of a medical emergency. The child must, of course, conform to all school policies about inappropriate cell phone usage during class.

Workplace Accommodations

Adults dealing with POTS symptoms will likely have an associated illness or broader form of dysautonomia that will affect their working status.

In the United States disabled individuals who are qualified for a position and want to work are granted an equal opportunity to do so under the 1990 Americans with Disabilities Act (ADA).

Under the ADA, a disability is defined as a physical or mental impairment that substantially limits a major life activity. These include, but are not limited to:

- caring for oneself
- performing manual tasks
- seeing
- hearing
- eating
- sleeping
- walking and/or standing
- sitting
- reaching
- lifting and/or bending
- speaking
- breathing
- learning
- reading

- concentrating / thinking
- communicating / interacting with others
- working

The legislation also covers the operation of a major bodily functions, including the immune system, sense organs, skin, digestion, bowel, bladder, brain, respiratory, circulatory, cardiovascular, neurological, endocrine, hemic, lymphatic, musculoskeletal and reproductive.

Many adult dysautonomia patients experience qualifying symptoms like those affecting manual labor requiring sitting or standing for extended periods or office jobs that call for intensive cognitive processing. These are only two examples of the many ways in which dysautonomia could contribute to workplace disability.

The law requires employers to provide a "reasonable accommodation." Some examples might be:

- Being allowed time off for medical treatment.
- An increased number of work breaks.
- Ergonomic seating.
- Lighting adjustments.
- Temperature adjustments.
- Access to foods, liquids, and medicines at all times.
- Extra time on assignments that have no crucial fixed deadline.
- Telecommuting opportunities during symptomatic periods.

Employers do not always have to provide the requested accommodation, and are free to choose among all available accommodations that would be effective. If the accommodation poses an undue hardship the employer may not be required to fulfill the provision, and they are not required to purchase any personal use items for their employees like compression stockings.

Understand that individuals are not required by law to disclose their disabilities. While it is a personal choice to discuss your dysautonomia with your employer, it can be to your advantage. If, for instance, you work in a government position, federal agencies strictly adhere to the letter of the law, and you may receive even more accommodations than you think you require.

If you believe that you are being discriminated against on the job due to your dysautonomia, contact your local office of the U.S. Equal Employment Opportunity Commission or visit the EEOC website at www.eeoc.gov.

POTS and Insurance

Under the best of circumstances, navigating the language of a health insurance plan is confusing and often discouraging. If you are investigating the extent of your coverage or negotiating with your company, you are looking for provisions regarding "Autonomic Nervous System Testing" or similar phraseology.

Most companies include caveats like "when it is medically necessary" or enumerate conditions for which the testing is acceptable like diabetic neuropathy, amyloid neuropathy, Sjogren's syndrome, idiopathic neuropathy, pure autonomic failure, and multiple system dystrophy.

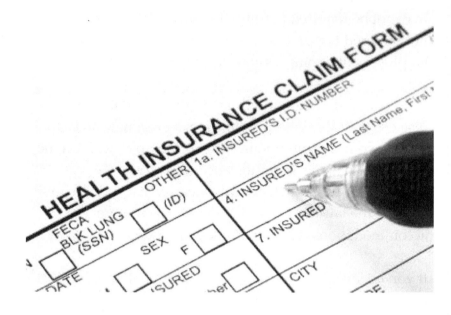

Even if the policy does not list POTS per se, be on the look out for passages that read along these lines, "Differentiate the diagnosis between certain complicated variants of syncope from other causes of loss of consciousness." You will know you are absolutely covered if you see a phrase like, "differentiate the cause of postural tachycardia syndrome."

Be aware, however, that insurance coverage is not set in stone. In October 2013, one of the largest insurance companies in the United States, WellPoint, discontinued coverage for autonomic testing. Other insurers, while not denying the coverage outright, require pre-certification or pre-approval for the coverage to apply.

You can still have the test if you are not given the go-head by your insurer, but you will be responsible for the cost. As discussed earlier in the text, some of the primary diagnostic tests used for POTS include:

- Posture Study
- Head Up Tilt Table
- Cardiac Output
- Beat-to-Beat Blood Pressure
- Valsalva maneuver
- Sinus Arrhythmia
- Transcranial Doppler
- Cold Pressor Test
- QSART Testing
- Endothelial Function

Always ask your doctor/hospital for a schedule of fees to help you decide what costs you can bear if it becomes necessary to do so.

POTS and Social Security

For older patients, Social Security disability payments are possible for POTS or other dysautonomic disorders but such illnesses are not the specific subject of a Social Security Administration (SSA) listing.

It will be necessary for the SSA to determine if your symptoms prevent you from working. This will require a careful review of the relevant medical records and a residual functional capacity assessment (RFC).

The SSA combines the RFC with a review of your past job

skills, education, and age to determine if there are other jobs you can safely and successfully preform.

To learn more about Social Security disability, visit the Administration's homepage at www.ssa.gov.

Part 5 – Research and Resources

Research into dysautonomic conditions including POTS is a field ripe with potential. Patients themselves can help by signing up for the POTS Research Registry at DysautonomiaInternational.org.

Working with ResearchMatch and funded by the National Institutes of Health, this effort will help to connect healthy volunteers with researchers. (The registry is only open to participants living in the United States.)

The purpose of the registry is to collect data on POTS patients to spur additional research efforts and to better understand the causes of the disorder to more effectively target successful maintenance and treatment.

As you begin to explore the world of POTS research, some notable names and efforts will immediately stand out.

Ongoing Research, Dr. Philip Low

Dr. Philip A. Low, who coined the acronym POTS in 1993, remains a leading researcher in the field of autonomic dysfunction. Some of his publications on the topic include:

- "A prospective, 1-year follow-up study of postural tachycardia syndrome." Kimpinski K, Figueroa JJ, Singer W, Sletten DM, Iodice V, Sandroni P, Fischer PR, Opfer-Gehrking TL, Gehrking JA, Low PA. Mayo Clin Proc. 2012 Aug;87(8):746-52.

- "Decreased orthostatic adrenergic reactivity in non-dipping postural tachycardia syndrome." Figueroa JJ, Bott-Kitslaar DM, Mercado JA, Basford JR, Sandroni P, Shen WK, Sletten DM, Gehrking TL, Gehrking JA, Low PA, Singer W. Auton Neurosci. 2014 Oct;185:107-11.

- "Effect of pregnancy on postural tachycardia syndrome." Kimpinski K, Iodice V, Sandroni P, Low PA. Mayo Clin Proc. 2010 Jul;85(7):639-44.

- "Gastric emptying in postural tachycardia syndrome: a preliminary report." Park KJ, Singer W, Sletten DM, Low PA, Bharucha AE. Clin Auton Res. 2013 Aug;23(4):163-7.

- "Midodrine Efficacy in Orthostatic Hypotension." Singer W, Joyner MJ, Sandroni P, Benarroch EE, Fealey RD, Mandrekar J, Low PA. J Gen Intern Med. 2014 Sep 9.

- "Orthostatic intolerance without postural tachycardia: how much dysautonomia?" Parsaik AK, Singer W, Allison TG, Sletten DM, Joyner MJ, Benarroch EE, Low PA, Sandroni P. Clin Auton Res. 2013 Aug;23(4):181-8.

- "Postural orthostatic tachycardia syndrome and general anesthesia: a series of 13 cases." Rabbitts JA, Groenewald CB, Jacob AK, Low PA, Curry TB. J Clin Anesth. 2011 Aug;23(5):384-92

- "Postural tachycardia in children and adolescents: what is abnormal?" Singer W, Sletten DM, Opfer-Gehrking TL, Brands CK, Fischer PR, Low PA. J Pediatr. 2012 Feb;160(2):222-6.

- "Postural tachycardia syndrome (POTS)." Low PA, Sandroni P, Joyner M, Shen WK. J Cardiovasc Electrophysiol. 2009 Mar;20(3):352-8.

- "Postural Tachycardia Syndrome associated with peripartum cardiomyopathy." Kimpinski K, Iodice V, Low PA. Auton Neurosci. 2010 Jun 24;155(1-2):130-1.

- "Preventing and treating orthostatic hypotension: As easy as A, B, C." Figueroa JJ, Basford JR, Low PA. Cleve Clin J Med. 2010 May;77(5):298-306.

An Autoimmune Connection?

In January 2014 the *Journal of the American Heart Association* published an article originally presented at the 24th International Symposium on the Autonomic Nervous system in Kohala, Hawaii in October 2013 and then at the Annual Scientific Session of the American Heart Association in November 2013 in Dallas, Texas.

Entitled, "The Autoimmune Basis for Postural Tachycardia Syndrome," the work was authored by the following researchers: Hongliang Li, MD, PhD; Xichun Yu, MD; Campbell Liles, BS; Muneer Khan, MD; Megan Vanderlinde-Wood, MD; Allison Galloway, MD; Caitlin

Zillner, BS; Alexandria Benbrook, BS; Sean Reim, BS; Daniel Collier, BS; Michael A. Hill, PhD; Satish R. Raj, MD; Luis E. Okamoto, MD; Madeleine W. Cunningham, PhD; Christopher E. Aston, PhD; David C. Kem, MD.

The abstract for the article reads, "Background Patients with postural tachycardia syndrome (POTS) have exaggerated orthostatic tachycardia often following a viral illness, suggesting autoimmunity may play a pathophysiological role in POTS. We tested the hypothesis that they harbor functional autoantibodies to adrenergic receptors (AR)."

(Adrenergic receptors are present on the surface of many of the body's cells and act like antennae to pick up signals from chemicals called catecholamines, particularly epinephrine and noepinephrine. The message tells the receptor to perform an action, like constrict a blood vessel or increase heart rate.)

The researchers identified a group of autoantibodies in some POTS patients that seem to directly influence heart rate. Their data supports the theory that some forms of POTS may be autoimmune in nature. If so, the condition could be managed with drugs that block key autoantibody activity while allowing the key receptors to remain "open" and functional. Since the findings were limited to only 14 patients with POTS, a larger controlled study is required to verify their findings.

For a more detailed discussion of this research see:
"New Evidence of Autoimmunity in POTS!" The Dysautonomia

Dispatch: The Blog of Dysautonomia International at: www.dysautonomiainternational.org/blog/wordpress/new-evidence-of-autoimmunity-in-pots/.

This research has generated so much interest in the dysautonomia community that Dysautonomia International in cooperation with researchers at Vanderbilt University and the University of Oklahoma created a POTS Antibodies Research Fund.

They met their initial research goal of $50,000 in two months. The fund remains open for other researchers interested in pursuing this line of study.

To learn more about the effort, to donate, and to review the appropriate 501(c)(3) non-profit status of the effort visit www.DysautonomiaInternational.org. Click on the link for "Donate/Shop."

Vanderbilt Autonomic Dysfunction Center

The Vanderbilt Autonomic Dysfunction Center, established in 1978, specializes in research, training, and patient care for all autonomic nervous systems disorders.

One of the preeminent researchers at the Center, Dr. Satish R. Raj, Associate Professor of Medicine and Pharmacology, is also a member of the Dysautonomia International Medical Advisory Board.

In advocating participation in the POTS Research Registry maintained by the group, Dr. Raj said, "[c]linical research is going to be the vehicle for advancing our understanding of POTS, and for the development of more effective therapies. ResearchMatch will allow for POTS researchers to more easily find those POTS patients interested in participating in research studies. I hope that ResearchMatch will catalyze our research."

Dr. Raj's paper "The Postural Tachycardia Syndrome (POTS): Pathophysiology, Diagnosis & Management" is considered a "must read" for POTS patients and their doctors. [Indian Pacing Electrophysiol J. 2006 Apr-Jun; 6(2): 84–99. Published online Apr 1, 2006.]

The entire text of the article can be accessed free of charge at www.ncbi.nlm.nih.gov/pmc/articles/PMC1501099/.

The lecture "POTS – A World Tour" presented by Dr. Raj at the 2013 Dysautonomia Patient Conference on July 6, 2013 can be viewed at vimeo.com/72346576.

Address for correspondence:
Satish R Raj MD MSCI
AA3228 Medical Center North,
Vanderbilt University
1161 21st Avenue South
Nashville, TN, 37232-2195, USA
Email: satish.raj@vanderbilt.edu

Other Leading Researchers

Other prominent researchers in the field of dysautonomia and POTS include:

- Dr. Peter Rowe from Johns Hopkins. His presentation "Dysautonomia and Postural Orthostatic Tachycardia in the Chiari/EDS Population" can be viewed at: vimeo.com/71903707

- Dr. Stephen Vernino at UT Southwestern Medical Center. His presentation "Autoimmune Autonomic Failure: A Treatable Under-diagnosed Condition" can be viewed at vimeo.com/32792885

- Dr. Paola Sandroni at the Mayo Clinic. Her presentation "Introduction to the Autonomic Nervous System and Overview of Autonomic Disorders" can be viewed at http://vimeo.com/73113927

Finding a Doctor

Finding a doctor with an understanding of POTS can often be frustrating. In your search for a physician, a good beginning resource is the Dysautonomia Information Network Physician List at: www.dinet.org/index.php/physician-list

Doctors are listed alphabetically by last name, but each column of the list can be sorted, so it's possible to group doctors by city or state as well as specialty. In the "Illnesses Treated" column, the acronym POTS is clearly visible even with a casual scan of the information. The page also contains a direct search form.

Since POTS is often caused by an underlying autonomic

disorder, consultations with physicians specializing in autonomic disorders are often necessary. See the membership listings at the American Autonomic Society at americanautonomicsociety.org to begin your search if your own doctor has no referral suggestions.

Survey of Recent Research

POTS is associated with so many corollary conditions that researching the illness can be an open-ended project. I have tried to pull together my notes into a coherent narrative with a "guide" style.

However, I do realize that many of you may want to dig deeper if your particular case does not fit the parameters outlined in this text.

For that reason, I am including a partial survey of the recent academic publications on POTS covering the years 2012-2014 with citations to help you locate the material on your own should you so desire.

―――――――

Abed, Howraa, Patrick A Ball, and Le-Xin Wang. "Diagnosis and Management of Postural Orthostatic Tachycardia Syndrome: A Brief Review." *Journal of Geriatric Cardiology: JGC* 9, no. 1 (2012): 61.

Adamec, Ivan, David Ozretić, and Mario Habek. "Autonomic Dysfunction in Multiple Sclerosis Presenting With Postural Orthostatic Tachycardia." *Acta Neurologica Belgica* (2013): 1–3.

Adamec, Ivan, Mila Lovrić, Dinka Žaper, Anabella Karla Barušić, Ivo Bach, Anamari Junaković, Antonija Mišmaš, and Mario Habek. "Postural Orthostatic Tachycardia Syndrome Associated With Multiple Sclerosis." *Autonomic Neuroscience* 173, no. 1 (2013): 65–68.

Arnold, Amy C, Luis E Okamoto, André Diedrich, Sachin Y Paranjape, Satish R Raj, Italo Biaggioni, and Alfredo Gamboa. "Low-Dose Propranolol and Exercise Capacity in Postural Tachycardia Syndrome a Randomized Study." *Neurology* 80, no. 21 (2013): 1927–33.

Bagai, Kanika, Candy I Wakwe, Beth Malow, Bonnie K Black, Italo Biaggioni, Sachin Y Paranjape, Carlos Orozco, and Satish R Raj. "Estimation of Sleep Disturbances Using Wrist Actigraphy in Patients With Postural Tachycardia Syndrome." *Autonomic Neuroscience* 177, no. 2 (2013): 260–65.

Bayles, Richard, KN Harikrishnan, Elisabeth Lambert, Emma K Baker, Alex Agrotis, Ling Guo, Jeremy BM Jowett, Murray Esler, Gavin Lambert, and Assam El-Osta. "Epigenetic Modification of the Norepinephrine Transporter Gene in Postural Tachycardia Syndrome." *Arteriosclerosis, Thrombosis, and Vascular Biology* 32, no. 8 (2012): 1910–16.

Benarroch, Eduardo E. "Postural Tachycardia Syndrome: A Heterogeneous and Multifactorial Disorder." Mayo Clinic Proceedings 87(12), no. 12 (2012): 1214–25.
Blitshteyn, S. "Postural Tachycardia Syndrome Following Human Papillomavirus Vaccination." *European Journal of*

Neurology 21, no. 1 (2014): 135–39.

Brewster, Jordan A, Emily M Garland, Italo Biaggioni, Bonnie K Black, John F Ling, Cyndya A Shibao, David Robertson, and Satish R Raj. "Diurnal Variability in Orthostatic Tachycardia: Implications for the Postural Tachycardia Syndrome." *Clinical Science* 122, no. 1 (2012): 25–31.

Busmer, Lorna, Lesley Kavi, and John West. "Postural Tachycardia Syndrome." *British Journal of Cardiac Nursing* 7, no. 5 (2012): 206–12.

Cases, Representative and Comorbidities in POTS. "Postural Tachycardia Syndrome." *Autonomic Neurology* 86 (2014): 89.

Chelimsky, Gisela, Shaista Safder, and Thomas Chelimsky. "Fgids in Children Are Associated With Many Nonpsychiatric Comorbidities: The Tip of an Iceberg?" *Journal of Pediatric Gastroenterology and Nutrition* 54, no. 5 (2012): 690–91.

Coffin, Samuel T, Bonnie K Black, Italo Biaggioni, Sachin Y Paranjape, Carlos Orozco, Phillip W Black, William D Dupont, David Robertson, and Satish R Raj. "Desmopressin Acutely Decreases Tachycardia and Improves Symptoms in the Postural Tachycardia Syndrome." *Heart Rhythm* 9, no. 9 (2012): 1484–90.

Deng, Wenjun, Yanling Liu, Angie Dong Liu, Lukas Holmberg, Todd Ochs, Xueying Li, Jinyan Yang, Chaoshu Tang, Junbao Du, and Hongfang Jin. "Difference Between Supine and Upright Blood Pressure Associates to the Efficacy of Midodrine on Postural Orthostatic Tachycardia Syndrome (Pots) in Children." *Pediatric Cardiology* 35, no. 4 (2014): 719–25.

Farmer, Adam D, Asma Fikree, and Qasim Aziz. "Addressing the Confounding Role of Joint Hypermobility Syndrome and Gastrointestinal Involvement in Postural Orthostatic Tachycardia Syndrome." *Clinical Autonomic Research* 24, no. 3 (2014): 157–58.

Gamboa, Alfredo, Luis E Okamoto, Satish R Raj, André Diedrich, Cyndya A Shibao, David Robertson, and Italo Biaggioni. "Nitric Oxide and Regulation of Heart Rate in Patients With Postural Tachycardia Syndrome and Healthy Subjects." *Hypertension* 61, no. 2 (2013): 376–81.

Gibbons, Christopher H, Istvan Bonyhay, Adam Benson, Ningshan Wang, and Roy Freeman. "Structural and Functional Small Fiber Abnormalities in the Neuropathic Postural Tachycardia Syndrome." *PloS one* 8, no. 12 (2013): e84716.

Giesken, Brittany and Miranda Collins. "A 46-year-old Woman With Postural Orthostatic Tachycardia Syndrome." *Journal of the American Academy of Physician Assistants* 26, no. 5 (2013): 30–32.

Green, Elizabeth A, Vidya Raj, Cyndya A Shibao, Italo Biaggioni, Bonnie K Black, William D Dupont, David Robertson, and Satish R Raj. "Effects of Norepinephrine Reuptake Inhibition on Postural Tachycardia Syndrome." *Journal of the American Heart Association* 2, no. 5 (2013): e000395.

Heyer, Geoffrey L, Erin M Fedak, and Aggie L LeGros. "Symptoms Predictive of Postural Tachycardia Syndrome (Pots) in the Adolescent Headache Patient." *Headache: The Journal of Head and Face Pain* 53, no. 6 (2013): 947–53.

Jarjour, Imad T and Laila K Jarjour. "Low Iron Storage and Mild Anemia in Postural Tachycardia Syndrome in Adolescents." *Clinical Autonomic Research* 23, no. 4 (2013): 175–79.

Jarjour, Imad T. "Postural Tachycardia Syndrome in Children and Adolescents." Seminars in pediatric neurology 20(1), no. 1 (2013): 18–26.

Jiménez-Cohl, Pedro, NM Earle, BR González, and EJ Thieck. "[Postural Orthostatic Tachycardia Syndrome (Pots): Report of 15 Cases]." *Revista Medica de Chile* 140, no. 2 (2012): 145–52.

Joyner, Michael J. "Standing Up for Exercise: Should Deconditioning be Medicalized?" *The Journal of Physiology* 590, no. 15 (2012): 3413–14.

Kanjwal, Khalil, Bilal Saeed, Beverly Karabin, Yousuf Kanjwal, Mujeeb Sheikh, and Blair P Grubb. "Erythropoietin in the Treatment of Postural Orthostatic Tachycardia Syndrome." *American Journal of Therapeutics* 19, no. 2 (2012): 92–95.

Kanjwal, Khalil, Bilal Saeed, Beverly Karabin, Yousuf Kanjwal, and Blair P Grubb. "Use of Methylphenidate in the Treatment of Patients Suffering From Refractory Postural Tachycardia Syndrome." *American Journal of Therapeutics* 19, no. 1 (2012): 2–6.

Katz, Ben Z, Julian M Stewart, Yukiko Shiraishi, Cynthia J Mears, and Renee Taylor. "Orthostatic Tolerance Testing in a Prospective Cohort of Adolescents With Chronic Fatigue Syndrome and Recovered Controls Following Infectious Mononucleosis." *Clinical Pediatrics* 51, no. 9 (2012): 835–39.

Khurana, R. "Postural Tachycardia Syndrome (Pots): What Do Palpitations Tell?" *NEUROLOGY* (2013):

Khurana, Ramesh K. "Visceral Sensitization in Postural Tachycardia Syndrome." *Clinical Autonomic Research* 24, no. 2 (2014): 71–76.

Kimpinski, Kurt, Juan J Figueroa, Wolfgang Singer, David M Sletten, Valeria Iodice, Paola Sandroni, Philip R Fischer, Tonette L Opfer-Gehrking, Jade A Gehrking, and Phillip A Low. "A Prospective, 1-Year Follow-Up Study of Postural Tachycardia Syndrome." Mayo Clinic Proceedings 87(8), no. 8 (2012): 746–52.

Kurozumi, A, Y Okada, K Nishida, S Yamamoto, H Mori, T Arao, and Y Tanaka. "[a Case of Postural Orthostatic Tachycardia Syndrome (Pots) With Difficulties in Differentiation From Hypoglycemic Attack]." *Journal of UOEH* 34, no. 4 (2012): 353–61.

Lewis, I, J Pairman, G Spickett, and JL Newton. "Clinical Characteristics of a Novel Subgroup of Chronic Fatigue Syndrome Patients With Postural Orthostatic Tachycardia Syndrome." *Journal of Internal Medicine* 273, no. 5 (2013): 501–10.

Li, Hongliang, Xichun Yu, Campbell Liles, Muneer Khan, Megan Vanderlinde-Wood, Allison Galloway, Caitlin Zillner, Alexandria Benbrook, Sean Reim, and Daniel Collier. "Autoimmune Basis for Postural Tachycardia Syndrome." *Journal of the American Heart Association* 3, no. 1 (2014): e000755.

Liao, Ying, Jinyan Yang, Fengwen Zhang, Stella Chen, Xueqin Liu, Qingyou Zhang, Yi Ai, Yuli Wang, Chaoshu Tang, and Junbao Du. "Flow-Mediated Vasodilation as a Predictor of Therapeutic Response to Midodrine Hydrochloride in Children With Postural Orthostatic Tachycardia Syndrome." *The American Journal of Cardiology* 112, no. 6 (2013): 816–20.

Light, AR, L Bateman, D Jo, RW Hughen, TA Vanhaitsma, AT White, and KC Light. "Gene Expression Alterations At Baseline and Following Moderate Exercise in Patients With Chronic Fatigue Syndrome and Fibromyalgia Syndrome." *Journal of Internal Medicine* 271, no. 1 (2012): 64–81.

Mitsufuji, T. "Csf Leakage Might be a Cause of Postrural Tachycardia Syndrome (Pots)." *CEPHALALGIA* (2013): Mustafa, Hossam I, Satish R Raj, André Diedrich, Bonnie K Black, Sachin Y Paranjape, William D Dupont, Gordon H Williams, Italo Biaggioni, and David Robertson. "Altered Systemic Hemodynamic and Baroreflex Response to Angiotensin Ii in Postural Tachycardia Syndrome." *Circulation: Arrhythmia and Electrophysiology* 5, no. 1 (2012): 173–80.

Nakao, Ryota, Hidetaka Tanaka, Kimitaka Takitani, Mitsugu Kajiura, Naoyuki Okamoto, Yukiko Kanbara, and Hiroshi Tamai. "Gnb3 C825t Polymorphism is Associated With Postural Tachycardia Syndrome in Children." *Pediatrics International* 54, no. 6 (2012): 829–37.

Nijs, J and K Ickmans. "Postural Orthostatic Tachycardia Syndrome as a Clinically Important Subgroup of Chronic Fatigue Syndrome: Further Evidence for Central Nervous System Dysfunctioning." *Journal of Internal Medicine* 273, no. 5 (2013): 498–500.

Nwazue, Victor C and Satish R Raj. "Confounders of Vasovagal Syncope: Postural Tachycardia Syndrome." *Cardiology Clinics* 31, no. 1 (2013): 101–9.

Ocon, Anthony J, Zachary R Messer, Marvin S Medow, and Julian M Stewart. "Increasing Orthostatic Stress Impairs Neurocognitive Functioning in Chronic Fatigue Syndrome With Postural Tachycardia Syndrome." *Clinical Science* 122, no. 5 (2012): 227–38.

Park, Ki-Jong, Wolfgang Singer, David M Sletten, Phillip A Low, and Adil E Bharucha. "Gastric Emptying in Postural Tachycardia Syndrome: A Preliminary Report." *Clinical Autonomic Research* 23, no. 4 (2013): 163–67.

Peggs, Kiffany J, HoVan Nguyen, Diba Enayat, Nancy R Keller, Ayman Al-Hendy, and Satish R Raj. "Gynecologic Disorders and Menstrual Cycle Lightheadedness in Postural Tachycardia Syndrome." *International Journal of Gynecology & Obstetrics* 118, no. 3 (2012): 242–46.

Plash, Walker B, Andre Diedrich, Italo Biaggioni, Emily M Garland, Sachin Y Paranjape, Bonnie K Black, William D Dupont, and Satish R Raj. "Diagnosing Postural Tachycardia Syndrome: Comparison of Tilt Testing Compared With Standing Haemodynamics." *Clinical Science* 124, no. 2 (2013): 109–14.

Popatia, Rizwana and Meera Subramaniam. "An Interesting Case of Dysautonomia Presenting With Dyspnea." *Pediatric Pulmonology* 49, no. 3 (2014): E25–26.

Prinsen, Hetty, I Jolanda M de Vries, Ruurd Torensma, Jeanette M Pots, Sasja F Mulder, Carla ML van Herpen, Lammy D Elving, Gijs Bleijenberg, Foekje F Stelma, and Hanneke WM van Laarhoven. "Humoral and Cellular Immune Responses After Influenza Vaccination in Patients With Chronic Fatigue Syndrome." *BMC Immunology* 13, no. 1 (2012): 71.

Raj, Satish R. "Postural Tachycardia Syndrome (POTS)." *Circulation* 127, no. 23 (2013): 2336–42.

Ross, Amanda J, Marvin S Medow, Peter C Rowe, and Julian M Stewart. "What is Brain Fog? An Evaluation of the Symptom in Postural Tachycardia Syndrome." *Clinical Autonomic Research* 23, no. 6 (2013): 305–11.

Ross, Amanda J, Anthony J Ocon, Marvin S Medow, and Julian M Stewart. "A Double-Blind Placebo-Controlled Cross-Over Study of the Vascular Effects of Midodrine in Neuropathic Compared With Hyperadrenergic Postural Tachycardia Syndrome." *Clinical Science* 126, no. 4 (2014): 289–96.

Schofield, JR, S Blitshteyn, Y Shoenfeld, and GRV Hughes. "Postural Tachycardia Syndrome (Pots) and Other Autonomic Disorders in Antiphospholipid (Hughes) Syndrome (Aps)." *Lupus* 23, no. 7 (2014): 697–702.

Seligman, William H, David A Low, Masato Asahina, and Christopher J Mathias. "Abnormal Gastric Myoelectrical Activity in Postural Tachycardia Syndrome." *Clinical Autonomic Research* 23, no. 2 (2013): 73–80.

Shibata, Shigeki, Qi Fu, Tiffany B Bivens, Jeffrey L Hastings, Wade Wang, and Benjamin D Levine. "Short-Term Exercise Training Improves the Cardiovascular Response to Exercise in the Postural Orthostatic Tachycardia Syndrome." *The Journal of Physiology* 590, no. 15 (2012): 3495–505.

Singer, Wolfgang, David M Sletten, Tonette L Opfer-Gehrking, Chad K Brands, Philip R Fischer, and Phillip A Low. "Postural Tachycardia in Children and Adolescents: What is Abnormal?" *The Journal of Pediatrics* 160, no. 2 (2012): 222–26.

Sousa, Alexandra, Ana Lebreiro, João Freitas, and Mª Júlia Maciel. "Long-Term Follow-Up of Patients With Postural Tachycardia Syndrome." *Clinical Autonomic Research* 22, no. 3 (2012): 151–53.

Stewart, Julian M, Marvin S Medow, Zachary R Messer, Ila L Baugham, Courtney Terilli, and Anthony J Ocon. "Postural Neurocognitive and Neuronal Activated Cerebral Blood Flow Deficits in Young Chronic Fatigue Syndrome Patients With Postural Tachycardia Syndrome." *American Journal of Physiology-Heart and Circulatory Physiology* 302, no. 5 (2012): H1185–94.

Wallman, Daniel, Janice Weinberg, and Anna Depold Hohler. "Ehlers–danlos Syndrome and Postural Tachycardia Syndrome: A Relationship Study." *Journal of the Neurological Sciences* 340, no. 1 (2014): 99–102.

Wang, Xiao-Li, Tian-You Ling, M Cristine Charlesworth, Juan J Figueroa, Phillip Low, Win-Kuang Shen, and Hon-Chi Lee. "Autoimmunoreactive Iggs Against Cardiac Lipid Raft-Associated Proteins in Patients With Postural Orthostatic Tachycardia Syndrome." *Translational Research* 162, no. 1 (2013): 34–44.

Wang, Xiao-Li, Qiang Chai, M Cristine Charlesworth, Juan J Figueroa, Phillip Low, Win-Kuang Shen, and Hon-Chi Lee. "Autoimmunoreactive Iggs From Patients With Postural Orthostatic Tachycardia Syndrome." *PROTEOMICS-Clinical Applications* 6, no. 11-12 (2012): 615–25.

Yang, Jinyan, Juan Zhao, Shuxu Du, Die Liu, Chunhin Fu, Xueying Li, Stella Chen, Chaoshu Tang, Junbao Du, and Hongfang Jin. "Postural Orthostatic Tachycardia Syndrome With Increased Erythrocytic Hydrogen Sulfide and Response to Midodrine Hydrochloride." *The Journal of Pediatrics* 163, no. 4 (2013): 1169–1173. e2.

Yun, Dong Joo, Han Na Choi, and Gun-Sei Oh. "A Case of Postural Orthostatic Tachycardia Syndrome Associated With Migraine and Fibromyalgia." *The Korean Journal of Pain* 26, no. 3 (2013): 303–6.

Zhang, Fengwen, Xueying Li, Chen Stella, Li Chen, Ying Liao, Chaoshu Tang, Hongfang Jin, and Junbao Du. "Plasma Hydrogen Sulfide in Differential Diagnosis Between Vasovagal Syncope and Postural Orthostatic Tachycardia Syndrome in Children." *The Journal of Pediatrics* 160, no. 2 (2012): 227–31.

Zhang, Qingyou, Ying Liao, Chaoshu Tang, Junbao Du, and Hongfang Jin. "Twenty-Four-hour Urinary Sodium Excretion and Postural Orthostatic Tachycardia Syndrome." *The Journal of Pediatrics* 161, no. 2 (2012): 281–84.

Zhang, Qingyou, Xia Chen, Jiawei Li, and Junbao Du. "Clinical Features of Hyperadrenergic Postural Tachycardia Syndrome in Children." *Pediatrics International* (2014): Öner, Taliha, Baris Guven, Vedide Tavli, Timur Mese, Murat Muhtar Yılmazer, and Savas Demirpence. "Postural Orthostatic Tachycardia Syndrome (Pots) and Vitamin B12 Deficiency in Adolescents." *Pediatrics* 133, no. 1 (2014): e138–42.

Škerk, Vedrana, Hrvoje Pintarić, Diana Delić-Brkljačić, Zvonimir Popović, and Hrvoje Hećimović. "Orthostatic Intolerance: Postural Orthostatic Tachycardia Syndrome With Overlapping Vasovagal Syncope." *Acta Clinica Croatica* 51, no. 1 (2012): 93–95.

Part 6 – Medical Definitions

Much of the terminology associated with dysautonomia, POTS, and the required testing is dense and confusing. I have included the following definitions to help you interpret what you are reading and being told by doctors.

adrenergic receptors – Receptors on the surface of cells that pick up signals from chemicals called catecholamines, particularly epinephrine and noepinephrine. The message tells the receptor to perform an action, like constrict a blood vessel or increase heart rate.

arrhythmias - Irregularity in the beating of the heart.

autoantibody – An antibody or protein produced by the immune system that reacts to the body's own tissues, cells, or cell components rather than to an outside "invader."

autonomic nerves - Nerves that regulate involuntary functions.

autonomic nervous system - Controls those body functions that do not require conscious thought including heart rate, blood pressure, and digestion among others.

Autonomic Reflex Screen - A variety of tests to assess blood pressure, heart rate, and sweating among other factors to judge the functioning of the autonomic nervous system.

bradycardia - A heart rate that is abnormally low.

brain fog - See cerebral hypoperfusion.

cardiogenic - Caused by the heart.

cerebral hypoperfusion - Confusion or "brain fog."

central nervous system - The brain and spinal cord.

deconditioning - Being out of shape after an injury or illness necessitating prolonged bed rest.

diastolic - The bottom number of a blood pressure reading.

dysautonomia - An umbrella term for several malfunctions of the autonomic nervous system including POTS (Postural Orthostatic Tachycardia Syndrome).

electromyography (EMG) - A test to check the health of muscles and nerves by inserting small needles into the muscles through which electrical pulses are transmitted and measured.

exercise intolerance - An inability to exercise without negative symptoms surfacing.

gastrointestinal - Relating to the stomach and/or digestive tract.

heterogeneous - Having many possible causes.

hypertension - High blood pressure, generally considered 130/90 or higher. (Please note that there are many considerations on what constitutes a "normal" blood pressure.)

hypotension - Low blood pressure, generally considered 90/60 or lower.

hypovolemia - Decreased volume of circulating blood.

idiopathic - Of unknown origin.

insomnia - An inability to fall asleep or to stay asleep that is chronic and affects day-to-day functioning.

Joint Hypermobility Syndrome - A benign syndrome that often exists in concert with POTS in which the patient's joints move beyond the normally expected range.

Nerve Conduction Velocity - A test that uses brief electric shocks to test the speed of electrical signals through a nerve.

neurally mediated neurocardiogenic - Caused by an interaction of the nervous and circulatory systems.

Neurocardiogenic Syncope - A brief loss of consciousness caused by a drop in both blood pressure and heart rate causing decreased blood flow to the brain. Also known as Vasovagal Syncope.

orthostatic - Being in an upright position, standing.

orthostatic hypotension - Abnormally low blood pressure that occurs when a person stands.

orthostatic intolerance - Adverse reactions when standing upright from a sitting or horizontal position.

pallor - Characterized by extreme paleness or loss of color.

parasympathetic nerves - Nerves that work while the body is at rest and under normal conditions. They decrease heart rate and stimulate digestion.

pathophysiology – The disordered physiological process seen in instances of disease or injury.

peripheral nervous system - The nerves that branch outward from the brain and spinal cord.

platelet aggregation - The clumping of platelets in blood as part of the process of coagulation.

pooling - When blood or fluids collect in the lower portions of the body.

postural - Referring to a position of the body, for example lying, sitting, or standing.

pulmonary circulation - Carries deoxygenated blood away from the heart and to the lungs for oxygenation before returning the blood to the heart.

somatic nerves - The nerves that regulate the movement of skeletal muscles.

splanchnic circulation - Consists of three vascular beds comprised of the stomach, pancreas, small intestine, and colon.

stroke volume - The amount of blood ejected by the heart with each beat.

supine - Lying down on the back.

sympathetic nerves - Nerves that control "fight or flight" reactions by increasing heart rate, constricting blood flow in the peripheral arteries, and raising blood pressure.

syncope - The experience of fainting or losing consciousness.

systemic - Affecting the whole body.

systolic - The top number in a blood pressure reading.

tachycardia - Elevated or racing heart rate.

tilt table - A motorized table on which a patient, braced against a foot support, can be placed at any angle between lying down and upright.

tremulousness - Uncontrollable and involuntary shaking.

varices - Enlarged veins.

vasoconstriction - Contraction or narrowing of the blood vessels.

vasodilation - Widening of the blood vessels.

Vasovagal Syncope - A brief loss of consciousness caused by a drop in both blood pressure and heart rate causing decreased blood flow to the brain. Also known as Neurocardiogenic Syncope.

venous - Pertaining to the veins.

venous pooling - The accumulation of blood due to gravitational pull.

Afterword

Clearly POTS symptoms can present under a wide variety of circumstances. For young people, especially those who have just experienced a rapid growth spurt, the syndrome is "developmental" in nature and can be managed until it passes with age and maturity.

In other cases, however, the syndrome is linked to an underlying condition that may or may not be correctable. In those instances, patients may face a lifetime of managing their POTS symptoms, including seeking the necessary accommodations to gain an education and hold a job.

Without question, all patients cope with a challenging medical climate in which very few doctors understand or have even heard about POTS. As you will read in the first-person accounts on blogs and in discussion forums, an endless round of tests and wrong conclusions generally prefaces a diagnosis of POTS.

This is what happened with my niece and on more than one occasion both she and her family were terrified with diagnoses of truly horrible diseases that in the end she didn't have. Such moments put you in the odd position of being both incredibly grateful and angry and frustrated with the medical bureaucracy all at the same time.

As I stated in the Foreword, I am not a doctor, nor do I intend for any of the information in this book to be taken as medical advice. My goal here has been to collate the information I amassed into an accessible format to help people first learning about POTS jumpstart their own personal education with this syndrome.

All POTS cases are unique, so "definitive" answers are often quite elusive. I have attempted to survey the circumstances under which POTS can surface and to talk about diagnostic testing, management, treatment techniques, and ongoing research.

My hope is that this information will be of use to families and individuals working to thread their way through the maze of medical information to arrive at practical and effective solutions. Because work with POTS and POTS awareness is ongoing, I encourage you to use what you have learned here as a stepping off point for ongoing research.

Like many "invisible" illnesses, POTS is often deeply misunderstood, especially when it occurs in otherwise healthy young people. It was with no small degree of outrage that I learned that a doctor archly informed my sister that Sylvie was just "lazy and wants to be the center of attention."

Far from it! My niece just wanted to get back to normal, which for her meant a full slate of activities with her friends and top-notch grades. POTS kept her away from her regular life for the better part of a year and a half before an accurate diagnosis allowed her to get the help she needed.

The fact that she did not fall behind in school and immediately took back up her life as her health began to improve makes the doctor's suggestion that she was a hypochondriac all the more infuriating.

POTS is a real condition that significantly effects the quality of life of any patient regardless of age. If you believe that you or a loved one suffer from this condition, stand up for yourself and insist that you be given the right tests by doctors knowledgeable in this condition and its management.

As is the case with many lesser known illnesses, you are your own best health advocate and may well know more than the doctors attempting to treat you!

Relevant Websites

Jodi Epstein Rhum
www.facebook.com/jodi.epsteinrhum

POTS & OI Recovery
www.potsrecovery.com

Dysautonomia International Blog
www.dysautonomiainternational.org/blog/wordpress/new-evidence-of-autoimmunity-in-pots/

AHA Journal - Clinician Update - Postural Tachycardia Syndrome
www.circ.ahajournals.org/content/117/21/2814.full

Dysautonomia Information Network Physician List
www.dinet.org/index.php/physician-list

New York Medical College
www.nymc.edu/fhp/centers/syncope/pots.htm

Pediatric Cardiology Center of Oregon
www.pccoforegon.com/blog/overview-of-pots-syndrome

POTS UK
www.potsuk.org

Vanderbilt Autonomic Dysfunction Center
http://www.mc.vanderbilt.edu/root/vumc.php?site=adc

Postural Orthostatic Tachycardia Syndrome - POTS
http://heartdisease.about.com/od/syncopefainting/a/Postura
l-Orthostatic-Tachycardia-Syndrome-Pots.htm

POT Syndrome
(POTS, Postural Orthostatic Tachycardia Syndrome)
http://www.medicinenet.com/pot_syndrome/article.htm

The Children's Hospital of Philadelphia
http://www.chop.edu/service/cardiac-center/heart-
conditions/postural-orthostatic-tachycardia-syndrome.html

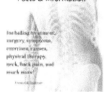

ISBN: 978-0-9896584-8-5

ISBN: 978-1-941070-01-7

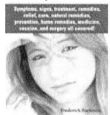

ISBN: 978-1-941070-02-4

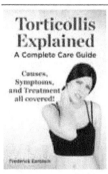

ISBN: 978-1-941070-05-5

Made in the USA
Las Vegas, NV
09 March 2023

68795132R00069